When God & Cancer Meet

when
GOD & cancer
meet

True stories of hope and healing

Lynn Eib

Tyndale House Publishers, Inc. • Carol Stream, Illinois

Library of Congress Cataloging-in-Publication Data

Eib, Lynn.
    When God & cancer meet : true stories of hope and healing / Lynn Eib.
        p. cm.
    Includes bibliographical references.
    ISBN-13: 978-0-8423-7015-8 (pbk.)
    ISBN-10: 0-8423-7015-3 (pbk.)
    1. Cancer—Patients—Religious life.   2. Cancer—Religious aspects—Christianity.   I. Title: When God and cancer meet.   II. Title.
    BV4910.33 .E37 2002
    248.8'6196994—dc21   2002002543

Printed in the the United States of America

12   11   10   09   08   07   06
12   11   10   9   8   7

dedication

This book is dedicated

with a heart full of praise to God;

with a heart full of love to my

husband, Ralph, & my daughters,

Danielle Joy, Bethany Noelle,

& Lindsey Michelle;

and with a heart full of gratitude to

Marc & Elizabeth Hirsh.

table *of* contents

acknowledgments

IT IS BOTH awesome and humbling to look back and see how the hand of God has brought me to the place where this book can be in your hands today.

I want to say **THANK YOU**:

To my parents, Bob and Gaynor Yoxtheimer, who gave me life, love, and a journalism degree and who always have been my biggest fans.

To all the cancer survivors and family members of cancer patients who let me write about their encounters with God so that others might find hope.

To all the members, past and present, of my Cancer Prayer Support Group, who remain in my prayers often and my heart always.

To my church family at Christ's American Baptist, whose prayers and acts of service got my family and me through my cancer ordeal and whose continued support upholds my ministry to cancer patients.

To oncology nurse Ruth Sieck, whose "laughter therapy" during chemo treatments blessed me and continues to bless others.

To my author-friend David Biebel, who convinced me to write this book and helped me get the process started.

To my writing buddy, Karen Yingling, who talked me into going to a writer's conference, where I got just the right contact name for Tyndale House.

To my acquisitions editor, Jan Long Harris, who believed in my message and was willing to take a chance on a first-time book author.

To my manuscript editor, Lisa Jackson, whose pen improved my book and whose prayers will increase its impact for the Kingdom.

introduction

WHEN I WAS in the hospital after my cancer surgery, a friend came into my room and told me God was going to teach me great things through this trial. I wanted to take the IV out of my arm, stab it in hers, and tell her, "You get in the bed and learn great things from God, because I don't want to learn this way."

If you or someone you love has been diagnosed with cancer, I doubt you're rejoicing over the possibilities of what you can learn through suffering. But I hope you are praying and believing that God can touch you. Whoever you are. Right where you are:

Newly diagnosed and in shock, praying there's been some mistake.

Facing surgery, praying the doctor can get it all.

Trudging through chemotherapy and radiation, praying they work.

Undergoing tests, praying for some good news finally.

Dealing with a recurrence, praying it's been found soon enough.

At the end of medical hope, praying for a little more time.

Holding the hand of a loved one, praying to be strong for them.

Whatever "cancer category" you fit into, this book has been written especially for you. It's the kind of book I wish I had read when I was diagnosed with advanced colon cancer at the age of thirty-six. Suddenly I was thrown into another world, a world I scarcely knew existed—the world of cancer—and I desperately needed some hope and encouragement.

Don't get me wrong; many people tried to give me hope and encouragement. They said things like, "You'll get through this," or "It'll be okay." But I wanted to scream back at them, "How do you know? You've never been through this!"

The first person to really give me hope was a woman named Pat who came up to me after my first hospital cancer-support-group meeting, put her arm around me, walked me to my car, and told me I would make it through my chemotherapy.

Do you know why I believed her? Not because she had years of medical training or decades of worldly wisdom. I believed her because she sported a brightly colored scarf on her head, still bald from chemotherapy. I knew that she knew because she had been there.

Pat was the first cancer survivor I ever knew personally. Now my life is filled with cancer survivors because I've spent the intervening years both as a volunteer cancer-support-group facilitator and as an employed patient advocate in my oncologist's office.

I have held the hands of hundreds of people with cancer, listened to the fears in their hearts, and seen what gave them hope. I know that cancer patients and their caregivers are longing for encouragement as they try to make sense of what might seem like senseless suffering. It is my prayer that this book will bring you that encouragement.

All the stories in this book are true, though a few names and details have been changed to protect the privacy of individuals or families involved. All the people in this book have been touched by cancer. But, more importantly, God has touched every person in this book in what I believe to be a miraculous way during his or her crisis with cancer. Sometimes God took the cancer out of them and sometimes He took them out of the cancer. But always, always, He touched them with His divine love and met their deepest needs.

It is my prayer that as you read these stories, you will experience God's peace and power and presence as never before. I pray that you will believe God can be trusted to meet your deepest needs because you can see His faithfulness in these people's lives.

You can believe their stories because they have been there.
You can believe me because I have been there.
You can believe God because He promises He *will* be there.

All the stories have what I consider to be "happy" endings, even though you may shed a tear or two as you read them. I know how important it is to hear stories of hope when you are facing cancer. People used to come up to me and tell me gruesome stories about their uncle who had the same kind of cancer I did and just "wasted away" or their grandmother who was "wracked with pain." I hated hearing these stories, but at first I tried to be polite and listen and smile.

Finally, I decided I could take it no longer and when people started a cancer story, I would interrupt them, smile, and say, "Does this story have a happy ending? Because if it doesn't, I don't want to hear it."

That reply really stopped people in their tracks, and I didn't have to listen to any more hopeless cancer stories. Every story in this book is a hope-filled story, even though not all of the individuals I describe were cured (on this earth) of their cancer. Each person found what he or she needed not to be defeated by cancer. None of them faced a hopeless end, but instead each found endless hope.

I have purposely chosen to write about people who faced extraordinarily difficult circumstances so that if your cancer journey is "easier" than theirs, you won't doubt that God can give you what you need. And if your journey is as difficult as theirs . . . well, you won't doubt God can give you what you need.

This is not a book of formulas that promise if you do this or don't do that, your prayers will be answered just the way you want them to be. I know such books exist because cancer patients and their families often want to talk with me when such a formula doesn't work for them.

This is a realistic book. It's real because it admits that some people get cured of cancer and some don't. It's real because it acknowledges there are no easy answers to the unfairness of life. It's real because it doesn't pretend that your faith in God will keep hard times away.

But it's also real because it shows real people, trusting in a real God in real life, who found real joy, real peace, real hope, real strength, and real encouragement.

It's real because it shows what can happen when God and cancer meet.

If you don't want to be defeated by cancer—no matter what it does or has done to you or your loved one, this is a book for you.

I hate the term *cancer victim*. It somehow implies cancer is the victor. It wins; we lose. That has not been my experience with cancer patients. While we can do little to choose whether we get cancer, we can do a lot to choose whether we are its victims. I don't just mean whether we live or die. I mean how cancer affects us in the deepest parts of who we are. I believe cancer cannot conquer our spirit unless we choose to become victims.

When I was diagnosed with cancer, I had personally known only two people with cancer. Now as a patient advocate for my oncologist—tending to the emotional and spiritual needs of his cancer patients and their caregivers—I know hundreds of people, most of whom I consider personal friends, who are fighting this dreaded disease. (As I write this, I just met my thousandth newly diagnosed cancer patient at our office last week.)

I have seen in my own life and in theirs that nothing, including conquering cancer, is impossible with God. I've seen how God has taken the worst tragedy of my life and turned it into my greatest triumph.

Even if you think it's impossible for God to turn your trial with cancer into a triumph, I pray you'll keep reading this book. It's not a book of advice for cancer patients and their caregivers. If you're like I was, you're already getting far too much advice from well-meaning people.

I don't like to give advice to people with cancer, even though it's my job to help cancer patients. My goal each work-day is to love people affected by cancer and move them closer to God, who truly can meet all their needs. I would never dream of suggesting that God is going to work in your life exactly as He did in mine or in any of the lives of other people in this book. He's far too big to be boxed in like that. But He will work in your life—in His perfect way and time.

I wish we could meet over a cup of coffee or tea so I could just listen to your story and pray with you and let God do the rest. But since this one-way conversation is the best we can do for now, grab a cup of coffee or tea, read these stories, and let God do the rest.

"God, You are making a really big mistake here."

HAD YOU SEEN me that late June morning in 1990, you would have thought me the picture of perfect health. Dressed in soft yellow, with my waist-length brown hair glistening in the summer sun and my smile radiating the deep happiness I felt, I was sure the colonoscopy test would confirm only a diagnosis of ulcerative colitis.

After all, I was only thirty-six. I didn't smoke or drink. I had exercised faithfully for several years, and I ate like a health nut. I had attributed occasional blood in my stool to an old pregnancy hemorrhoid and the occasional bowel irregularity to something I had eaten.

But when the gastroenterologist came to my bedside in outpatient surgery with the results of the procedure, both my husband Ralph and I knew immediately that something was wrong.

"We found a tumor," he said, simply.

With those four words, my world turned upside down. There was a pause that seemed to last forever. No one spoke, and no one looked at anyone else.

"Do you think it's cancer?" I finally blurted out.

The doctor nodded affirmatively as his eyes filled with tears.

I can still see Ralph's ashen face as he stood at the end of the hospital gurney. This was his worst nightmare revisited. Some twenty years earlier, when Ralph was only a newlywed, a doctor had diagnosed his first wife with amyotrophic lateral sclerosis (Lou Gehrig's disease), which is incurable.

"No!" I yelled, over and over, as if somehow the force of my words could make this nightmare not true. I sobbed and sobbed, eventually hyperventilating. The doctor motioned to the nurse to give me more intravenous sedative. I kept thinking how all the nurses would go home and tell their families about the patient who "lost it" today.

But I didn't really care what they thought. After all, I was the one with cancer. And my tears were the only way to express my feelings at that moment—for me, for our three daughters, and for my husband. Though as a journalist, words were my business, no words could fully capture the moment. *Shocked* and *devastated* were too mild. It was as if someone had hit me between the eyes with a brick and I was afraid to get back up for fear they would hit me again.

I had never given cancer a second thought. No one in my immediate family or our very large extended family had battled the "Big C." Some of my friends seemed constantly worried about getting cancer, including one who often called me with her "lump of the month" story.

But not me. I had been confident it wasn't going to happen to me. *People with cancer look sick or at least feel sick, don't they?* And, after all that Ralph had endured already, could such a serious disease strike another spouse? The odds were against it. Weren't they?

"Do you have a surgeon?" the gastroenterologist inquired.

"No," I muttered. *Do people have surgeons in the same way they have hairdressers?* "I've only been in the hospital to give birth."

He said he would arrange a consult.

The half-hour ride home was the longest and quietest of our sixteen years of married life. There was nothing my husband could have said to make me feel any better, unless he could have told me that the entire thing had been a terrible mistake, the diagnosis a lie.

Five days later I had surgery to remove the tumor and resection the colon. I was told that if the cancer had been caught in the early stage, I would be considered cured and need no further treatment. But if it had advanced to the lymph nodes or beyond, I would have at best a 50 percent chance of surviving with the help of chemotherapy and/or radiation.

I begged God for the former. I endlessly explained to Him why that would be so much better.

Three days later, at 7 A.M., the surgeon and his resident delivered the pathology report. I could tell from their body language that the news wasn't good. They stood against the wall at the end of my hospital bed, as far away from me as they could get and still be in the same room.

"Cancer was found in five of twenty lymph nodes," the surgeon explained matter-of-factly. "You will need chemotherapy and radiation."

Again I cried, but no one moved toward me to comfort me.

"Have you ever known anyone who underwent chemotherapy?" he asked, seeming to grasp for words in order to continue the conversation.

I nodded, recalling a fourteen-year-old girl who had died from bone cancer and a young mother who had died with a brain tumor. Their images flooded my mind. Again, I hyperventilated.

Still, neither doctor moved toward me, but instead the surgeon called a nurse to help me breathe into a little paper bag. How I wished the doctor had at least held my hand for a moment or just patted my shoulder and told me that this was not an automatic death sentence.

"Do you want me to call your husband?" the doctor asked, still at the foot of my bed. I nodded between sobbing gasps into my little brown bag.

Now I was really frightened. I desperately needed Ralph. But, for whatever reason, the surgeon did not call him. So for three hours I lay in the room thinking about what it was going to be like to have chemotherapy pour through my veins. I had a little conversation with myself as I tried to control my weeping.

Get a grip on yourself, my head told my heart. *What are you so afraid of? Nausea and vomiting? You were sick night and day for six months with all three of your pregnancies. Mouth sores? You've had them before. Needles? You're not afraid of them. Losing your hair? It'll grow back. Don't be so vain,* my head stated matter-of-factly. But my heart didn't buy it. I just cried harder as I stroked the hair that I desperately wanted to keep.

Yes, that's what I'm afraid of, I admitted. *I don't want to look sick for my children and my husband. I can't imagine watching my hair fall out.* I disliked the vanity of my feelings, but it was how I felt.

I finally called Ralph at 10 A.M. I was shaking so badly my voice was barely audible, and he kept asking me to repeat everything.

"It's bad," I told him. "I need you right away."

I couldn't even get my lips to form the word *chemotherapy.* The fear of facing that, for me, was worse than the initial shock of cancer.

Ralph arrived shortly. At about noon the surgeon strolled in and said he had just tried to call my husband but there was no answer. "By the way," he added, "did I mention that you won't lose your hair with the chemo?"

I didn't know whether to hug him or smack him.

Baldness or not, this nightmare was not going away. I became consumed with thinking about dying. Almost any personal question made me cry, especially anything that reminded me of our daughters, then eight, ten, and twelve years old. *Will I see them grow up? How will they make it without me?*

Lying in that bed, I had lots of time to talk with God, whom I thought had made a big mistake in my life. I told Him so in no uncertain terms. I knew the promise in the

Bible in Romans 8:28 that says He will cause all things to work together for good, but I also knew that this promise sometimes can take a while to happen, and I wasn't interested in waiting that long. I told God I didn't want Him to make something good come out of the nightmare unfolding before my eyes. Instead, I wanted Him to take it away.

"You are making a really big mistake here," I fumed. "There's absolutely nothing You can ever do to make up for this because it is too awful. And don't think You are going to pull me through this somehow and I'm going to go and minister to cancer patients, because I won't do it!"

I think He must have smiled at me like a knowing mother does with a rebellious toddler at bedtime.

Three weeks after surgery I started weekly chemotherapy with Dr. Marc Hirsh, an oncologist in Hanover, Pennsylvania. I had met Dr. Hirsh the previous summer when he had visited the church my husband pastors. More recently, we had renewed our acquaintance when I had done a feature story for the local newspaper about a new cancer support group at the hospital. I knew he was a Messianic Jew—a Jew who believed in Jesus (Yeshua) as the promised Messiah.

I wanted Dr. Hirsh and his faith on my healing team. I had no idea that I would one day end up on his healing team—but that's getting ahead in my story.

I had never really minded needles, but the chemo needle was a different story. My veins would move and the nurse would fish around inside my arm. I felt sick before the drugs even started. The drug combination I was getting was not as toxic as most chemo regimes. It usually took weeks for patients to feel any side effects, I was told.

Not so with me.

I felt sick from the onset, but the antinausea medicine made me so sleepy I couldn't function, so I chose to be sick instead. (Thankfully, antinausea drugs that don't cause drowsiness are now available!)

I developed mouth sores.
I was terribly fatigued.
My taste buds were shot.
I lost twenty pounds.

Even water made me nauseated, and the outside air smelled so bad some days that I had to hold my nose just to walk outside.

On top of all that, I was allergic to the main drug. My nose ran constantly and my eyes watered profusely. (The chemo scarred my tear ducts so severely that my right eye continues to water to this day despite two surgeries to correct the problem.)

The palms of my hands and the soles of my feet turned flame red and felt like they were on fire.

My joints swelled so much that I could hardly bend my fingers, and I had to walk on the sides of my feet some days.

Three times the skin peeled off my feet.

I experienced just about every possible side effect from the chemo. All the while, I knew that hundreds of people in sixteen states were praying for me. So, it seemed logical, at least to my emotional self, to ask God *why* everything was so hard.

"Why aren't things going easier for me?" I cried out. "Would it be too much to ask to feel normal again for just a couple of hours?" But I heard only silence from heaven.

At that time, the treatment for colon cancer was weekly for a year (with a break every few weeks). About five months into my treatments, I was driving to my oncologist's office and talking to God.

"I don't think I can take this anymore," I told Him. (I figured that since He knew even my thoughts, I might as well say them out loud and get them off my chest.)

"I've been praying to You and lots of people have been praying to make this easier on me, but it's getting worse. I'm not a quitter, so I'll keep going. But I don't know if I can take another seven months of this," I said as the salty tears rolled down my cheeks.

When I got into the doctor's office that day, he examined my hands and feet and said, "I don't think you can take much more of this. Let's get you through another month. I think if the chemo is going to work, it's had enough time to do so. Besides, I think the studies will eventually show that six months is enough for this treatment." (He was right—standard treatment for colon cancer is now only six months.) So I hung on, finishing my chemo in February 1991.

When I returned for my first checkup in May, I was the only person in the chemo room who wasn't there for a treatment that day. I knew I should feel happy that I had finished treatment, but I didn't. As I looked around that room of people in recliners hooked up to poles with saline-solution bags, I was overcome with sadness. Some of them looked so thin and ill, and others looked so tired and afraid. I began to weep.

I wanted to take away their pain, but I couldn't.
I wanted to give them peace, but I couldn't.

Then God spoke to my heart: "But you know the One who can, and you can tell them about Me."

"But I just want to put all this behind me and go on with my life," I argued. "Besides, I don't want to hang around people with cancer. It will be depressing and they'll die and I can't handle it. I won't do it."

A few weeks later, however, I came up with an idea that I figured would suit both God *and* me: I would start a cancer support group, and God would *have* to let me live because everyone in that group would need me!

But as I spent time each day praying to God, He reminded me that He doesn't play "Let's Make a Deal." He wanted me to get involved—no guarantees.

If you've ever sensed God wanted you to do something, but you were reluctant, you probably also know you didn't have any peace until you said yes.

Finally, like a pouting child, I gave in: "I'll do it, but I won't like it," I told Him, temporarily forgetting that my primary concern was to obey, and He would take care of the rest.

I started the Cancer Prayer Support Group in October 1991 with four people. My intent was to have a one-hour, once-a-month meeting. *That shouldn't be too depressing,* I figured.

But almost immediately I could see that the people coming to the group needed more support than that. Not only that, but I found that I actually felt *better* after the meetings rather than worse. So we started meeting twice a month and have been doing so ever since. And guess what soon became a great source of joy in my life—the support group! As the months rolled by, I secretly began to pray that I would be able to quit my job and volunteer with cancer patients full-time.

In July 1995, on the fifth anniversary of my cancer surgery, I told our congregation how God had blessed me through my cancer experience—through my friends in the support group and through Marc Hirsh and his wife, Elizabeth, who had become very close friends and prayer partners with my husband and me.

I concluded with this sentence: "Someday I hope I can quit my job and minister full-time, sharing God's peace and love with cancer patients."

I knew it was an unrealistic wish—there was no way financially that we could afford for me to quit my job and volunteer. But less than a year later, my prayer became a reality when Marc asked to meet with Ralph and me. He said he had been praying about something and felt it was the right time to ask.

"Would you join our clinical staff, ministering to the emotional and spiritual needs of our cancer patients and their families?" he said. "I will match whatever you're making at your present job."

I tried to sound very spiritual. "I'll pray about it," I said.

But Ralph gave me an incredulous look and said, "You've been praying about this for a year. Say yes!"

So since May 1, 1996, I have had a job where I listen to patients' hopes and fears, praying that God will heal them physically, emotionally, and spiritually. I ask Him to bless each one, and I believe that He will. I see cancer—or any illness or trial—as a very deep pit, but I believe that the love of God is deeper still. And the reason I believe this is because of—and not in spite of—my own experience with cancer, which God has transformed from an ordeal to a blessing to others.

In the year before my new job offer, I had been meditating on the Bible verse Ephesians 3:20 which speaks of our God "who is able to do immeasurably more than all we ask or imagine" (NIV).

There is no doubt in my mind that God has done far more in my life than I could ask or imagine, and I know that He can do that in your life too.

Do I think He's going to give you a job as a patient advocate for your oncologist? Probably not.

Do I think He is able to do something equally amazing in your life? You bet I do.

I can't tell you how, when, or where God will bring a blessing through your trial of suffering. But I can tell you why—because His Word promises He will. Romans 8:28 says, "And we know that God causes all things to work together for good to those who love God, to those who are called according to His purpose" (NASB).

God will bring blessing through your trial because you matter greatly to Him and He longs to show you that. He may bless you with physical healing, or He may bless you by healing you emotionally of some deep-seated hurts. He may bless you spiritually with the joy of knowing Him in a way you never have before. Or He may bless others through you in unimaginable ways.

My blessing from cancer is certainly *not* the one I sought, but because God knows me and loves me, He knew how to bless me.

He knows you. He loves you. He can bless through your trials . . . if you let Him decide the blessing.

Be encouraged: God wants to bring blessing through your cancer experience; you just need to let Him decide the blessing.

∼ Guy

Close Encounters of
the Divine Kind

"DOES YOUR FRIEND know he shouldn't be alive?"

I still remember exactly where I was standing when Marc posed that question to me concerning my friend Guy, a long-time member of the Cancer Prayer Support Group and a prostate-cancer survivor.

I wasn't sure why Marc would make such an assertion about my very healthy-looking, very much alive, very cancer-free friend, but it sure stopped me in my tracks.

"I don't think I've ever heard him mention that he was surprised to be alive," I responded tongue in cheek as we chatted in the tiny office stairwell just before Marc was ready to have a consult with Guy.

Then, turning serious, I asked, "So, why shouldn't he be alive?"

Guy, now a widower in his early seventies, had been diagnosed with prostate cancer in late 1993 and had undergone surgery, radiation, and hormone therapy. His PSA level (a blood test which can show the presence of prostate cancer) had been undetectable for years. I hadn't ever heard the particulars of Guy's diagnosis, but I figured the cancer had been caught soon enough and had been successfully treated. Guy was at our office on this day in June 1999 to see Marc concerning a non-cancer-related blood abnormality that had recently shown up on routine blood tests.

"He had Stage D prostate cancer," Marc said to me, still holding in his hands Guy's old medical records.

Now, if you've ventured very far into the world of cancer, you know that the stage of a cancer at diagnosis is very important and that nearly all Stage D—sometimes called Stage IV—cancers are not considered medically curable. (A few late-stage cancers, such as Hodgkin's, testicular, and thyroid, do have a good chance of being cured, and I personally know people who have been cured of each of these.)

Stage D prostate cancer, however, would not be on the list of those with a potential for medical cure.

But there it was in black and white in Guy's surgeon's notes dated January 25, 1994: "moderately differentiated adenocarcinoma of the prostate, Gleason 6, Stage D with metastasis to right pelvic lymph nodes."

A later dictation from a urologist confirmed again an "incurable pathology" and in oncology terms described Guy as having "margin-positive disease with positive right obturator lymph nodes as well." In plain English, they couldn't get it all.

It must have seemed quite clear to everyone involved at the time that Guy's cancer was not curable.

Everyone except Guy.

"I never knew my cancer was incurable," says Guy, insisting that he either wasn't told, or if he was, it never registered.

"When Dr. Hirsh told me that I had [been diagnosed in 1994 with] Stage D prostate cancer . . . Wow . . . I just couldn't believe it!" he recalls. "I looked at him and I said, 'You know Who healed me, don't you?'"

Guy doesn't know exactly when it happened. He doesn't know if it was a quick divine touch or if God somehow supernaturally increased the healing power of the various medical treatments he endured, but he gives all the credit for his survival to God.

"That day at Dr. Hirsh's, I knew for sure it was God who healed me, and I just felt so grateful to be alive," he says.

Obviously, finding out your cancer was incurable several years *after* you've been pronounced cured greatly alters the way you respond to that news! (Guy is definitely the only person I know who was *excited* to hear his cancer was Stage D.)

But excitement and gratitude were hardly the feelings he experienced in December 1993, when the cancer was first found.

At that time, cancer already was a very unwelcome intruder in his life.

Peg, his wife of thirty-four years, had died from a rare, inoperable cancer in September 1991, and his middle son, Mike, had completed chemo and radiation for testicular cancer in 1992.

Now it was Guy's turn.

"I didn't get angry," he recalls, "but I felt very empty and I said, 'Why, Lord, why?'"

Even though Guy had had a strong faith in God for twenty-some years before his diagnosis, it wasn't easy for him to face cancer without Peg at his side.

A radical prostatectomy was scheduled for late January 1994 and Guy remembers the anxious moments before he went under the surgeon's knife.

"Before I went into the OR, they prepped me, and Mike's minister was up to see me and he asked me if he could pray with me," Guy says. "Then they took me out of the room and down the hall.

"Before we got to the [operating room] door, I said, 'Stop!'" Guy recalls. "The guy pushing me said, 'What's wrong?' but I just told him again to stop.

"I looked up and pointed up and I said, 'Lord, You know me and I know You—do with me what You will,'" he remembers. "Once I said those words, I was so at peace and I said to the guy that was pushing me, 'Let's go!'

"I left [my cancer prognosis] up to God and I wasn't afraid of anything. I had a peace that I can't describe right."

I would describe what happened that moment as a close encounter of the divine kind.

As Guy reached out to God, he said a simple prayer of surrender, giving the Master of the universe permission to have His way in Guy's life. He did what I believe we all need to do: agree to let God simply be God.

> **Let Him be the unfalteringly faithful God, willing to strengthen us for any and every circumstance.**
> **Let Him be the incredibly sovereign God, wise enough to know how and when to answer any and every prayer.**
> **Let Him be the mighty awesome God that He is, powerful enough to heal us at any and every level—powerful enough to heal my friend Guy, body, mind, and spirit.**

That prayer on the way to the operating room wasn't the first such close encounter with God that Guy had—the first had happened years before when a coworker had challenged him to begin living for God—but it was the first of many more during his journey with cancer.

Another one came the day after he finished his thirty-ninth and final radiation treatment and was on his knees praying for God to spare the life of his youngest son, Dave, who was buried alive in a stone-filled silo at work. That divine encounter ended after eight hours with his son being rescued to the amazement of everyone, including the head of the rescue operation, who remarked afterward that Dave "shouldn't be alive."

When I decided to include Guy's story in this book, I knew that his body had been cured against all medical evidence and that his mind had been healed of worry and fear even though he had had to face cancer without his beloved wife. What I didn't know until I interviewed him was that God had used the Cancer Prayer Support Group to heal his spirit.

Guy admits that after his wife's diagnosis, he was angry. Peg was only sixty and was a hardworking woman who loved her family and her God very much.

"All through her radiation and chemo, she never missed a

day's work," he recalls. "She went to work at the sewing factory and then went to treatment. Even if she was sick in the night, she still went to work the next day.

"I was a little angry with God that she would get cancer," he says. "When she died, I felt so alone and was still angry with God for taking her."

Guy also admits that he had always had a hard time dealing with illness, and this became more difficult when cancer hit home.

"If anybody ever talked to me about being sick, I didn't like to hear about it and I would just turn it off," Guy explains. "Especially after Peg got cancer, I did not want to talk about it with anybody. I got real sour about it."

Sour is definitely not a word that those in our support group would use to describe Guy. Quite to the contrary, he's one of the most joyful people in our group and we can always count on him to give us a much-needed laugh.

He often shows up at group meetings wearing colorful wigs or "googly" glasses in case anybody has lost their hair and feels a little strange. Sometimes he walks in with his "disguise," while other times he sneaks it on when we're going around the table doing introductions. Either way, he has a wonderful sense of humor and he can always bring smiles to our faces.

When he was besieged with hot flashes during his hormone therapy, instead of being embarrassed by his flushed face and dripping brow, he used the frequent occurrences during our meetings to get us all laughing as we watched him giggling and fanning frantically. His openness and honesty are refreshing to newcomers and old-timers alike in the group.

But he remembers when he was a different Guy.

"I'll never forget when I came in there [to the support group] for the first time," he says. "I was scared to death.

"It was the first time in my life I ever opened up about hurting or being sick or anything else," he says. "Like I said, I just didn't talk about it.

"But you got me hooked," he says. "I talked about my wife and everything I was feeling and I just kept talking and talking. I never knew it would feel so good to talk about it all.

"Before I had cancer, if anyone talked about being sick, I didn't want to hear it," Guy says. "Now I'm more compassionate and I like to listen and see people smile and make them laugh.

"One thing I can't do is walk around with a long face anymore—the Lord has taken that away."

In those early days after my own cancer diagnosis, I wondered if I would ever laugh again. Two days before I went in for surgery, we took the girls to a movie as a treat to help get everyone's minds off what was ahead. The three of them laughed through one of the *Back to the Future* flicks, but I only brushed away my silent tears in the darkened theater.

If you or your loved one are still in those early dark-days-after-diagnosis, please remember they are just that.

Just as the Bible promises that "weeping may endure for a night, but joy comes in the morning" (Psalm 30:5 NKJV), so it is with a diagnosis of a life-threatening illness. The pain, fear, and sorrow that initially grip your mind and body won't last forever. You will smile again and even laugh again. The tears won't always flow so freely.

Even if you are facing a recurrence or a medically incurable cancer, I believe you can and will find joy again as you let God heal your wounded spirit.

Give yourself time to absorb all that has been thrown at you, and give God time to make something new and good from the shattered pieces.

Most importantly, don't run out ahead of God by trying to deal with all the endless negative possibilities facing you down the road. They are just that: possibilities.

Never forget we have a God who loves to do the improbable and specializes in the impossible—things like healing Guy of incurable cancer, filling him with peace when worry would have been so much easier, and turning his "sour" heart into a heart of joy.

I remember the first improbable thing God arranged for me within forty-eight hours of my cancer diagnosis.

That year I had been using the well-known devotional book *Streams in the Desert,* volume two, by Mrs. Charles E. Cowman. I had mentioned to my husband that the sometimes-archaic language and life situations described didn't seem to speak to my life. But when I start something, I usually finish it, so that year I continued to read the little book with dated daily readings each morning.

I was diagnosed with cancer on Tuesday, June 26. (You don't easily forget the day your world turns upside down.) On Thursday morning, before I went to meet my surgeon, I sat down to read my devotional. I did it because I knew it was the right thing to do, not because I felt like doing it. I was feeling alone and afraid, and I was wondering if my life was going to be cut short.

But the God of the improbable and, yes, even the impossible was about to meet me there.

The June 28 devotional was based on Psalm 23 and talked about how "goodness and mercy" will follow us all the days (good and bad) of our life because the Lord is our Shepherd and He cares for us, His sheep.

And then came the part where I encountered God: "This devotional thought may be read by someone who is being severely tested almost to the breaking point! Someone wondering about the tomorrows! He knows all about *your* tomorrows, and is thinking in advance for *you!* Yes, *for you!* For *you* He careth! Hide away in your heart the gracious promise: 'How precious are thy thoughts unto me, O God!'"[1]

I was crying so hard by the time I finished those short paragraphs that I could barely make out the words on the page.

God had somehow managed to take words written in the early 1900s and arrange for them to be on the right date to heal my spirit in 1990.

He gave me my very own stream in the desert.

I knew at that moment that God had what I needed to face my trial and, more importantly, He would give it to me at just the right time.

God knows if you are in the desert and He knows how to give you streams in the midst of it.

But it won't happen if you don't go to Him and *seek* an encounter with Him.

No matter where we are on our spiritual journey, if we seek Him, we will find Him. And the encounter we will have with Him will be unlike anything else we've ever experienced.

Just as thousands of years ago God promised the Israelites they would return from captivity in Babylon, I believe He promises us that we won't remain in the spiritual desert if we seek Him. He promises us that we will encounter Him and that He has divine plans for us.

"'For I know the plans that I have for you,' declares the Lord, 'plans for welfare and not for calamity to give you a future and a hope. Then you will call upon Me and come and pray to Me, and I will listen to you. And you will seek Me and find Me, when you search for Me with all your heart'" (Jeremiah 29:11-13 NASB).

I had an encounter with God on June 28, 1990, because by faith I went to Him.

I didn't really *feel* like reading that little book that day and seeking God. I would have rather just felt sorry for myself because the desert was so unfamiliar and so hot. But had I done that, I would have missed the refreshment God had for me—the healing stream he had for my weary, thirsting spirit.

Guy had an encounter with God as he paused to put his trust in God on the way to the operating room even though he didn't feel like he could face cancer again.

How is *your* walk in the desert going? Are *you* seeking God? I'm not asking whether you pray and ask God to heal the cancer. I'm assuming you do that.

I'm talking about something much more personal and life-changing. I'm talking about:

Going to His Word and expecting Him to meet you there.
Sitting in His presence and basking in His love for you.
Standing at His throne and waiting for His blessing
** for you.**
Coming to God and wanting Him in your life more
** than anything.**

It's in those kinds of moments that we truly encounter God and allow Him to begin His healing work in us, body, mind, and spirit. When we set aside our agenda, we can learn His agenda. When our voice is quiet, we can hear His quiet voice. When we take our eyes off ourselves, we can see Him so much more clearly.

I experienced my first postdiagnosis encounter with God when I read that devotional and knew the words were a direct message from the Almighty to me. I felt like a little child safe in the arms of her loving Father.

Nothing had changed, and yet everything had changed, because I had encountered God and His healing touch. I still had cancer and I still had to face surgery. I still didn't understand it all and I still didn't like any of it, but it was well with my soul.

I could join with the psalmist and say, "O Lord, my heart is not proud, nor my eyes haughty; nor do I involve myself in great matters, or in things too difficult for me. Surely I have composed and quieted my soul; like a weaned child rests against his mother, my soul is like a weaned child within me" (Psalm 131:1-2 NASB).

Many more such encounters followed during my battle with cancer as I continued to seek God and believed He would meet me wherever I was in my spiritual journey.

My friend Guy says his faith has never been stronger than

since he was diagnosed with cancer and began to have special close encounters of the divine kind. That's what happened to every other person I've written about in this book as well.

God had many kinds of healing in store for Guy—healing of his Stage D prostate cancer, healing of his anger over his wife's cancer, and healing of his "sour" heart, to name a few.

God has a lot of healing in store for you.

I hope you'll seek an encounter with Him (actually, many encounters) so you don't miss the healings—the wholeness, the blessings—He longs to give you.

"Now may the God of peace Himself sanctify you entirely; and may your spirit and soul and body be preserved complete, without blame at the coming of our Lord Jesus Christ. Faithful is He who calls you, and He also will bring it to pass" (1 Thessalonians 5:23-24 NASB).

Be encouraged: God's amazing power can heal you, body, mind, and spirit.

～ Susan

The Fear behind the Smile

I kNEW AS soon as I met Susan in September 1996 that we were going to be good friends.

She was a lot like I had been when I was diagnosed with cancer: young and afraid.

The difference was that in June of 1990, I didn't know anyone else young and afraid and facing cancer and chemotherapy. I didn't have anyone (on earth, at least), for a long time, whom I really felt understood what I was facing. I longed to know another young mother who had walked in similar shoes and could relate to my anxieties.

That's why when I meet certain cancer patients today, I know immediately we're going to be good friends because I can give them what nobody gave me for a long time: a friend who remembers what it feels like to be young and afraid and facing cancer.

By some standards, Susan and I probably had a rather strange friendship. We never had lunch together or went shopping or did the kinds of things that most friends do. We didn't share clothes or recipes, but we did share our hearts. Susan was really at the end of her rope when I met her. Shortly after we met, she committed herself to the local psychiatric hospital because of a deep depression. As she sat in her room locked away from the outside world, I don't think anybody—certainly not Susan—expected that God was going to use cancer to give her a peace and security she had never found in life before.

Susan had battled depression for years before discovering, at the age of forty-eight, that she had colon cancer and it had spread to the lung. I know it might sound unreal to those of you who often struggle with depression, but I don't think I had ever really been depressed in my whole life until I found out I had cancer. Many of my closest friends through the years, including my husband, have battled that dark cloud which can settle in seemingly for no reason and refuse to go away, but I never had.

Although I had never walked in Susan's shoes, I could imagine how it felt for someone like her, who already was struggling with depression, to be told she had something else to be depressed about: cancer.

It was this last straw that almost put her over the edge, and her husband, Steve, and I both wondered how she would ever deal with chemotherapy or anything else still down the road. I don't know all the things in Susan's life that played a part in her emotional struggles, but I do know cancer was not even at the top of the list. She had faced far worse things, including sexual abuse by a male neighbor that began at the age of eleven and continued until she married her husband, Steve, at sixteen.

I don't know what Susan looked like as an adolescent, but she was beautiful when I met her: tall and thin, with high cheekbones; long, wavy, reddish-brown hair; and a big, gorgeous smile. Steve later told me that her smile was often a cover-up for the pain and anger she felt inside—there was real fear behind the smile.

But Susan's diagnosis did *not* put her over the edge. In fact, ever so slowly, as she clung to the promises of God, she backed away from the edge and began to deal with things that she never before thought she could face. She and Steve started attending the Cancer Prayer Support Group, and soon she began encouraging newcomers there. In the chemo room at the office, Susan was a "regular," since she came in weekly for her two-hour treatment.

It didn't take long for her tender heart to be evident there, and she soon began to reach out to others, encouraging them with words of support that they, too, could face this battle. More than once another patient commented to me about the woman in the corner chair who was so nice. One patient described her as "the pretty one, you know, about thirty-five." I told him she had children almost that old, and he couldn't believe it. Susan and I had a good laugh over that one!

By this time Susan and I were praying together regularly, and she was looking to the Bible to find the strength she needed to face this life-threatening illness. It was obvious to me that her journey with cancer had become a spiritual trek.

Finally, in September 1997, just one year after we first met, that journey took an important turn. I remember the phone conversation clearly.

It was a Thursday, two days after our biweekly support-group meeting. I had done something at that meeting that I never had done there before—I had shared how I came to know God in a personal way while I was a sophomore at Ohio State University. I had told the group that I had discovered that faith was not about being religious but about having a relationship with God. I had said that that discovery had changed my life forever and had given me eternal life. I told them I would be happy to talk more about it with anyone who was interested.

So when Susan called, I knew why.

"I wanted to talk to you some more about what you said the other night," she said rather hesitantly. "I've always believed in God, but I don't think I have a personal relationship with Him."

"A lot of people are like that," I assured her. "They have a head-knowledge but not a heart-knowledge. They know about God, but they don't know Him personally. It's kind of like a famous person you've heard of and whom you believe exists, but that knowledge doesn't transform your life in any way."

"I went to a counselor one time," Susan said, "and she said I was a good person and hadn't done too many bad things and would go to heaven. Is that right?"

Since I don't have any counseling degrees and I don't ever want to suggest that my opinions are superior to those of others, I answered her with one of my favorite questions: "Do you want to know what the Bible says?"

I ask that question because I believe there are things that are absolutely true—not because you say so or I say so, but because God says so. So I shared with her what the Bible, God's Word, says about how we get to heaven:

We can't earn it by good works.
Jesus paid the price for our sins.
He is the only way to have peace with God.

"I really want to have peace with God, to know Him personally," Susan told me. I could tell by the urgency in her voice that she was very serious.

"What do I have to do?" she asked.

"It's a prayer away," I told her.

"Can I do it by myself, or does someone have to be here with me?"

"You don't need anybody but you and Jesus," I responded.

Then there was a long silence on the other end of the phone, and I sensed she was hesitant, but I wasn't sure why.

"We could even pray on the phone together if you want," I finally said.

She eagerly agreed. Now, I must tell you I have prayed with many people as they've put their trust in the Lord, but it has always been face-to-face, never over the phone. It felt a little strange, and I really wished I could reach out and hold her hand and see the tears that I knew were streaming down her beautiful face. But instead I pressed the receiver to my ear, closed my eyes tightly, and led her in a simple prayer of surrendering her life to God.

When we finished I told her the angels in heaven were rejoicing and so was I.

"Can I come to your church on Sunday?" she asked.

"Of course you can, and we'll sit together," I said, wishing she could see the tears streaming down my own face.

Did all of Susan's problems go away after that simple prayer? No. But her greatest problem did. She knew where she was going to spend eternity. And four days later, when she found out the cancer had returned, she knew that the Lord would be her Shepherd and walk with her through the valley ahead.

Shortly thereafter, Susan began another course of chemotherapy that temporarily shrank the tumors. As a result, she lived more than a year. At the last support-group meeting she attended, Susan was an incredible encouragement to another member named Jack, who had just found out his cancer was incurable (see chapter 7).

I was amazed as I watched Susan that night.

Could this be the same Susan who had just about gone over the edge two years before? Was this the same Susan who had been so depressed *before* she got cancer that she despaired of her life?

She looked the same on the outside (even with her wig), but she was far different inside. This new Susan sat and calmly told Jack that her cancer was incurable and it didn't seem like God was going to answer her prayer to be healed.

"But I've been thinking, and He's really answered a lot of my other prayers," she continued. Every eye in the room was riveted on her as she started naming those prayers.

Prayers that she would see her fiftieth birthday.
Prayers that she would see her oldest son's
house finished.
Prayers for a long-dreamed-of trip to Tennessee.
Prayers that she would see her only daughter married.
Prayers that she would hold her new grandson.

"He's answered all those prayers for me, and I didn't think any of those things could happen," she explained, wiping a tiny tear from the corner of her eye while still maintaining her composure.

I could see Jack and his wife, Jeannette, across the table, and I knew Susan's words were shedding light on their own struggle with unanswered prayers. I was so proud of her and what she did that night, truly encouraging them in a way I could not. Later they, too, would stop and think and recount all the prayers the Lord had answered for them.

Susan was especially excited at that last group meeting and wanted to share a note she had received in the mail that day from a stranger. The woman had heard from a relative about Susan's health struggles and wanted to tell Susan she was praying for her. (When a complete stranger sends a card just to let you know they're thinking of you or praying for you, it is an incredible blessing. It's one of the things I like to do now for people I will never meet, because I know how much it touched me.)

Inside the note to Susan was a little prayer card with a Bible verse and a picture of a stately, white lighthouse. As soon as she saw it, Susan said, she had started to cry. She loved lighthouses, but of course the stranger had no way of knowing that.

"I think God told her to give me that card," Susan told our group, as we all nodded in agreement.

Later Susan called the stranger and told her about her love for lighthouses.

"You know," the woman said, "I had a different card picked out for you and I was praying and felt God telling me to pick out the lighthouse one instead."

Whenever I see a lighthouse, I still think of Susan and how God sent her a personal message from Him via a stranger that day. I'm also reminded of how this beautiful woman who almost had her light snuffed out by the dark of depression became a light to other overwhelmed souls.

"Taking chemo not only changed Susan's life from day one,

but it changed my life as well," her husband, Steve, later wrote to me. "There are no words to describe what [you] did for the last two years of my wife's life before she went to meet Jesus."

I appreciate Steve's kind words, but the way I look at it, there are no words to describe what *God* did for his wife's life the last two years of her life. I know she felt His unconditional love in a never-before-experienced way and discovered a security and peace in Him that she didn't think was possible.

Before I met Susan, she felt that she had been given more in life than she could handle. Despite a devoted husband and four loving children, life was definitely overwhelming. One of the things that confused her was a popular statement she often heard people say. Maybe people say it to you. Maybe you've said it yourself:

God doesn't give you more than you can handle.

Does that ring a bell? I hear it a lot, especially from cancer patients or their family members who feel like they have more than they can handle. They usually say something like this: "Now, I know God doesn't give us more than we can handle, but . . ." Many people are under the misconception there is a Bible verse that states this fact.

There isn't.

The closest thing I can find is 1 Corinthians 10:13, which says, "No temptation has seized you except what is common to man. And God is faithful; he will not let you be tempted beyond what you can bear. But when you are tempted, he will also provide a way out so that you can stand up under it" (NIV).

I do believe that there is *never* a time we are tempted to sin when we simply have no choice but to give in. God always provides a way of escape so we can withstand temptation. The Bible also tells us that temptations do not ever come from God.

I also believe, however, that sometimes trials come into our life that *are* more than we can bear on our own, and cancer often is one of them. I believed Susan when she said that her difficulties were more than she could handle. I consider myself a strong person, but facing cancer and the fact that my possibility of dying was greater than my possibility of surviving made me feel very weak.

"This is more than I can handle," I remember telling God, trying not to sound too whiny.

"I know," He answered. "But it's not too much for Me."

That was one of the most freeing things I learned through my cancer journey. It was all right that I sometimes had more than I could handle. That's when I would see the Bible verse in Philippians 4:13 come true in my life: "I can do all things through Christ who strengthens me" (NKJV).

I didn't have to reach down inside myself and muster up some super strength. God supernaturally supplied it to me as I trusted in Him.

What a relief!
Even if my own resources were exhausted, God's would
  never be.
My strength might be sapped, but He could still move
  mountains.
Everything could be changing around me, but He was
  always my Rock.

During those first early dark-days-after-cancer, I often thought of the shepherd boy David as he went into battle against the giant Goliath. Do you know what his battle cry was? He wasn't like The Little Engine That Could, chugging along and repeating, "I think I can, I think I can."

No, I believe he was thinking, "I know I can't, I know I can't." He was the youngest and smallest boy in his family. Goliath was more than nine feet tall. But David's battle cry was, "I know God can, I know God can." If you read 1 Samuel 17:47 you'll hear his exact words: "The battle is the Lord's." That phrase appears many times throughout the Old Testament, and it was what I said to myself as I awoke on most postdiagnosis mornings.

"I feel like a little shepherd with a slingshot facing a giant named Cancer, and it is more than I can handle," I told the Lord. "But I am so glad it is not more than You can handle. The battle belongs to You, Lord. Fight for me and through me. Do what I cannot do on my own."

And He did.

Just like He did for Susan and for every other person in this book. Sometimes you may get more than you can handle in your own strength. That's okay. Whatever has happened to you has not taken God by surprise or caught Him off guard. He's prepared for the battle and will equip you with whatever you need *not* to become a victim of this giant called Cancer, but instead, to become a victor over it!

Be encouraged: Even though we sometimes may be given more than we can handle, we never will be given more than God can handle.

~ Lynn & Jane

When God Did the
Heimlich Maneuver

IF YOU'VE EVER been around children very long, you've probably heard them say, "That's not fair!" My own kids have said it *zillions* of times, sometimes daily during those trying teenage years. But if we're honest, I think it's not only children who want things to be fair. I think it's human nature for all of us to long for fairness . . . and that can make the diagnosis of cancer especially difficult.

You may feel it's unfair for you or your loved one to have cancer because you're too young, or you've taken such good care of your body, or you've hardly been sick a day in your life, or you've already had to face cancer with another relative, or you have enough other problems.

I really believed—and still do—that my colon cancer diagnosis was *very* unfair. My good diet, exercise, young age, and healthy living should have prevented it, but they didn't. Every doctor I met shook his head and said I had done everything right *not* to get cancer.

I don't know if I ever said it out loud, but I definitely thought it many times: *This is NOT fair.*

That's the way Lynn Myers felt too, when he was diagnosed with non–small cell lung cancer at the age of forty-eight. Lynn never smoked a day in his life, exercised just about every day, and had no family history of any cancer. The doctors were pretty surprised at the diagnosis. His two teenage sons were pretty shocked. And his wife, Jane, was pretty ticked.

Everybody agreed it was pretty unfair.

What nobody realized at the time was that Lynn's family was about to learn firsthand what it means not to confuse life with God.

"Being given the diagnosis of lung cancer and being a nonsmoker just didn't seem fair," Jane remembers. "It was a diagnosis we thought we'd never get, and I was angry.

"He was diagnosed at Christmas and that seemed especially hard," she recalls.

(I imagine there's a holiday you associate with your—or your loved one's—cancer diagnosis. I had surgery on July 2 and finally emerged from the fog of anesthesia two days later to sit on the bed, listening to fireworks in the distance and wishing I could watch my girls wave sputtering little sparklers in our driveway.)

The timing of the diagnosis in the life of Lynn's family also seemed especially unfair. They were on the brink of the long-awaited "empty nest," as their older son was a senior in college and their younger one a senior in high school. Two gradua-tions and their twenty-fifth wedding anniversary were all coming up within the next year.

"This should have been the time our children were leaving and we were going into the second half of our marriage," Jane says. "Lynn was looking forward to retiring sometime in the next eight to ten years and concentrating his life on some of his other interests.

"I know no time is a good time to get a cancer diagnosis, but it still just seemed such a bad time to get this news," she adds.

I met Jane and Lynn in February 1999, when he came in for his first chemo treatment at our office. We vaguely knew of each other because we had children in the same grades and we shared many mutual friends in our community. My first impressions of them were that she was really mad and he was really strong.

Jane says I was right on both accounts. Lynn was definitely the strong one in their relationship—strong physically, strong emotionally, and strong psychologically. He lifted weights every day in their home gym, often took three-mile runs around town, and practiced martial arts two or three times a week. He especially enjoyed relaxation and meditation and was one of those few people who could control his blood pressure and heart rate through breathing exercises.

But being a strong, disciplined, self-controlled person can have its disadvantages, too, as Lynn found out. He believed in God and was a regular church attender, but he was very self-reliant. Other than a few frightening times as a young marine in Vietnam, he had never really sought or experienced the power and presence of God in his life.

I remember when he finally did experience this power and how excited he was. It was June 10, 1999, and he called me at work early in the morning, obviously very thrilled.

"I've got to tell you what God did for me last night," he said as his words tumbled out in an uncharacteristically rapid manner.

I was rather surprised to hear him talking like that. First, Jane was the "talker" in the family and the one who usually called me. Second, Lynn was tough and didn't talk about what others did for him.

But things were different this morning.

"I wasn't feeling well all last evening," he told me. "I couldn't breathe, and I had to sit up in the recliner with the air conditioner and a fan blowing right on me so I could get enough air.

"I was so weak I couldn't even bend over to put on my socks," he said. "It felt like air just wasn't getting through to my lungs, and I was really scared—not about dying but about suffocating."

Why didn't you go to the emergency room or better yet call an ambulance? I thought as I listened to the description of his struggle to breathe. But then I remembered: *Lynn is a tough, self-controlled, disciplined man. He doesn't like to need things from other people, especially not for himself. He wants to take care of himself and others, too. Acknowledging weakness and asking for help just isn't his style.*

"So, what did you do?" I asked him.

Lynn said he had started praying at about 1:30 A.M.

Now, even though this religious man certainly had prayed before in his life, this prayer was different.

It was the prayer of a man who had nothing *but* a prayer.

"I started telling God I couldn't handle this on my own and I needed help, and I was asking Him to do something for me," Lynn said.

He didn't know it at the time, but Jane also was awake and praying the same earnest plea to God at the exact same time.

Within a few moments, Lynn coughed hard and then coughed again.

"Suddenly, I could breathe fine," he said. He lay down flat on the bed and slept peacefully for the rest of the night.

"I felt just like God had reached down and done the Heimlich maneuver on me!" he told me on the phone. "I never experienced anything like that! I know it was God who did that for me. It was amazing!"

I told him I never heard of God doing the Heimlich maneuver on anyone before, but since He is often called the Great Physician, I was sure He knew how!

When I hung up the phone after that conversation, I sat there almost in disbelief at the amazing way God can and does speak to us in our moments of deepest need. I knew Lynn would never be the same after that cough.

As the months went by and Lynn's disease managed to stay one step ahead of the chemo, he became very weak physically. But spiritually he had never been stronger. It was almost as if when the cancer drained him, it just left more room for God to fill him.

Once, near the end of Lynn's life, Jane shared with me how

much they had grown together spiritually since the diagnosis, even while fervent prayers were *not* being answered the way they had hoped. She had heard me tell the people in the support group many times not to be afraid of whatever was ahead because God would give them just what they needed, just when they needed it.

"You always said it could happen, but I couldn't imagine it really would for us," she told me.

Maybe you can't imagine it could happen for you or your loved one.

You can't imagine that you can be strong even while you're weak.
That you can have peace even while you're in turmoil.
That you can feel a quiet joy even when you're sad.
That you can experience God's faithfulness in the midst of life's unfairness.

You don't have to take me at my word or even Jane at her word. I do hope you'll take God at His word. Many times in His Word He promises us a supernatural presence through trials. I especially love Isaiah 43:1-2:

> *Fear not, for I have redeemed you; I have summoned you by name; you are mine. When you pass through the waters, I will be with you; and when you pass through the rivers, they will not sweep over you.* (NIV)

Jane and Lynn walked through deep waters—probably some of the deepest waters imaginable—but the flood did not overwhelm them. Instead, God took them through it and the whole time they felt His comforting presence.

"On the journey we walked, we really weren't afraid," Jane says. "I can honestly say there wasn't a time when Lynn was afraid, because he knew and felt God was there."

God was there in a special way during that time when life was unfair to them. He was especially faithful.

I don't know how deep your waters are. Maybe they're only ankle deep, but you're still really scared because you never learned to swim. Maybe they're waist deep and rising fast. Or maybe you're bobbing up and down, searching for something to help you stay afloat.

Perhaps you are crying out with the psalmist:

> *Save me, O God, for the waters have threatened my life. I have sunk in deep mire, and there is no foothold; I have come into deep waters, and a flood overflows me. I am weary with my crying; my throat is parched; my eyes fail while I wait for my God.* PSALM 69:1-3 NASB

No matter what your "water level" or your "swimming ability," I believe you need to learn the same lesson about fairness that Lynn and Jane did: Don't confuse life with God.

I should have learned this lesson a long, long time ago. After all, one of my parents' favorite phrases was, "Life's not fair."

I heard it plenty of times and I always hated hearing it. Nobody who is being treated unfairly wants to hear it. It tries to give a logical response to a heartfelt emotion. But as an adult I read something in a book by Philip Yancey that took that childhood truth one step further and forever changed how I looked at the fairness of life.

In Yancey's book *Disappointment with God,* he writes about a man named Douglas whom he interviewed because he thought Douglas might feel great disappointment with God. Life, as Yancey describes it, had been very unfair to Douglas. While his wife was battling metastatic breast cancer, Douglas was in a car accident with a drunk driver and suffered a terrible head injury that left him permanently disabled, often in pain, and unable to work full-time.

But when Yancey asked this victim of unfairness to describe

his disappointment with God, Douglas said he didn't feel any and instead told Yancey the following:

"I have learned to see beyond the physical reality in this world to the spiritual reality. We tend to think, 'Life should be fair because God is fair.' But God is not life. And if I confuse God with the physical reality of life—by expecting constant good health, for example—then I set myself up for crashing disappointment.

"If we develop a relationship with God *apart* from our life circumstances," said Douglas, "then we may be able to hang in there when the physical reality breaks down. We can learn to trust God despite all the unfairness of life."[1]

Cancer is very unfair. Even if you "did" something to "get" cancer or didn't do something *not* to get it, it's still unfair. Maybe you are a smoker diagnosed with lung cancer. Cancer is still unfair, because only about 20 percent of smokers develop lung cancer; 80 percent do not. Maybe you quit smoking twenty or thirty years ago and you still got cancer. Hardly fair.

Perhaps you didn't get regular mammograms, PAP smears, or PSAs, and now you have cancer. Guess what? It's still not fair, because lots of people don't get those screening tests and they don't get cancer. Besides, some people get them faithfully and the cancer isn't even detected! That seems even more unfair.

Go ahead and say it.
It's not fair that I have cancer.
It's not fair that my loved one has cancer.
It's not fair that this has happened to us right now.
Say it, but don't be confused that life should be fair
    because God is.
Life is not fair, but God is not life.

God is, of course, much bigger than life, and what He is doing in our life will truly change this life as well as ultimately transcend life itself.

Jane and Lynn saw and felt that many times during their "unfair" journey. Jane says God gave them an emotional strength that they not only felt but that others saw in them.

"It was interesting to hear the remarks of people who couldn't believe how we were handling things," Jane says. "I told them, 'That wasn't us, that was God coming through us.'"

God also gave them an understanding of life they hadn't embraced before.

"We saw that life had been unfair to others, too," Jane says.

That revelation came mostly after they became regular members of the Cancer Prayer Support Group.

"We realized we weren't the only ones who had been given this raw deal," Jane says, recalling all the great people they met at the support group. "In fact, there always seemed to be someone worse off than we were."

I think support groups can help us get over our own pity parties as we rub shoulders regularly with others who have received unfair news and have uncertain futures. In just our little group alone, I've seen plenty of examples of unfairness over the years.

I met Peggy and Nick, who married after both their spouses died only to have Peggy diagnosed with multiple myeloma a month after their wedding.

And Michelle and Jamie, in their twenties, who, six months after they said "I do," found out Michelle had Hodgkin's disease and later learned a bone marrow transplant would leave her unable to bear children.

And Doris, who just got her mantle cell lymphoma in remission, only to be diagnosed with another rare cancer, leiomyosarcoma.

And Steve, who was diagnosed with prostate cancer at the young age of forty-two and had two more recurrences by the time he was forty-five.

And Ron, whose mother and brother both died from cancer while he was fighting his own battle with colon cancer.

Each had to learn to distinguish between what life was handing them and what God was doing *in* them.

"We were such control people," Jane says. "We really had to learn about letting go and letting God."

Letting go of our wants and desires and letting God have His way is a lifelong struggle for all of us. I witnessed Lynn wrestling with this one day in the hospital's intensive care unit as we chatted. It was the only time I ever saw him cry throughout his cancer ordeal.

"All I want is to work and take care of my family," Lynn told me as tears filled his weary, hazel eyes. "That doesn't seem like too much to ask, does it?"

"No it doesn't," I responded as tears filled my eyes too. "I don't understand what God is doing—or even not doing—in your life right now," I told him. "The only thing I know to do is to walk by faith and not by sight. What we see doesn't make sense, but we can't see it all. Only God can. I trust Him that He will be faithful in this life and all things will be fair in the next life."

He nodded, and we prayed that he could feel in his heart what he knew in his head.

After that conversation and prayer, Lynn never got to work again as a draftsman at the local paper mill. He never got to take care of his family the way he wanted to. But his wife told me those final weeks together brought them a spiritual intimacy unlike anything they had ever experienced.

"The time I had with Lynn at the end was so special," she recalls. "We would sit and read Scripture together and share.

"Sometimes I would sit on the bed and read to him. I don't know the Bible really well, but I was always guided to the right place for God to speak to us."

She found verses such as Philippians 4:11: "I have learned to be content whatever the circumstances" (NIV).

And Romans 8:18: "I consider that our present sufferings are not worth comparing with the glory that will be revealed in us" (NIV).

And 2 Timothy 1:12: "I know the one in whom I trust" (NLT). Jane asked that the following quote from author Philip Yancey be read during Lynn's eulogy because it had encouraged them both so much when they read it:

> Every time a believer struggles with sorrow or loneliness or ill health or pain and chooses to trust and serve God anyhow, a bell rings out across heaven and the angels give a great shout. Why? Because one more pilgrim has shown again that he or she understands that Jesus is worth it all. God is faithful.[2]

The week before Lynn passed away, a visitor to his home remarked, "You are amazing; how do you keep going?"

Lynn's reply: "I know I can't carry this alone. You have to surrender and trust."

Difficult words for a man used to carrying his own weight. Difficult words for someone used to taking control of the situation. Difficult words for most of us. But they are the response God longs to hear when life is unfair.

There's a local law firm that advertises on the radio by spotlighting people who have had awful things happen to them and then hired a lawyer to rectify the situation. The commercial concludes that you, too, should call this law firm "when life hands you moments you just don't deserve."

I like Lynn's advice even better: When life hands you moments you just don't deserve, surrender to and trust in a faithful God.

Forever, O Lord, Thy word is settled in heaven. Thy faithfulness continues throughout all generations.

PSALM 119:89-90 NASB

Be encouraged: Even when life is unfair, God is faithful.

"We don't think she's going to make it."

I HOPE YOU are part of a cancer support group where you can share laughter and tears. I'm a firm believer—and scientific studies agree—that cancer patients tend to live longer and better when they regularly attend such a group.

Most of the people who come to our Cancer Prayer Support Group have medically incurable cancer. I didn't plan it to be a group like that, but it seems those are the people who need the most emotional and spiritual encouragement, so they tend to come to my group instead of the more traditional groups that concentrate on education and information about cancer.

This is a story about a member of our support group who, against all odds, survived her cancer ordeal.

Melissa came to my group because she's a Christian and wanted some encouragement as a newly diagnosed Hodgkin's lymphoma patient. She really didn't fit in, however, with the rest of the group for two good reasons: First, at only twenty years of age, she was a decade younger than anyone in the group. Second, diagnosed with a Stage IIA cancer and given an 85 percent chance of surviving, she had about double the cure odds of anyone else.

Everyone expected Melissa to breeze through her chemo in a few months, get a clean bill of health, and be off to the art school she had dreamed of since graduating from high school.

The odds were certainly in her favor. We were all glad that somebody in our group was definitely going to be okay.

But things didn't proceed according to plan. After the first round of chemo, the CT scan showed the tumors had shrunk, but not as much as normally would be expected. Marc still was cautiously optimistic that she could get a remission. Melissa went for radiation therapy, but within a month another CT scan showed the tumors were growing. She had resistant disease, Marc told me. That was really bad, he added.

Those once-promising odds of a cure were plummeting drastically.

He sent her to Johns Hopkins Hospital, about an hour away, to consult with doctors about a possible bone marrow transplant. The doctors agreed she was a good candidate for a transplant and at first thought there might be a 35 percent chance to cure her, but later they determined she had only a 15 percent chance she would be rid of Hodgkin's.

Her younger sister, Lynn, turned out to be a perfect match as her bone-marrow donor, and in December 1995, just days after her twenty-first birthday, Melissa was given a lethal dose of chemotherapy intravenously and then "rescued" from death with a transfusion of some of her sister's healthy bone-marrow cells. Obviously, it was a very risky procedure, but for patients like Melissa it was the only medical hope of a cure.

The bone marrow transplant went off without a hitch, and afterwards, Melissa and her mom moved into the outpatient quarters across the street. Doctors believe it's better for transplant patients not to be in the hospital, where there are all sorts of germs and where patients often grow lonely from the isolation. Instead, Melissa and her mom came over to the hospital briefly each day for Melissa to be checked.

Melissa felt so well that she didn't stay inside much. Instead, she donned her protective mask, climbed into her wheelchair, and went off for some fun. Often when I would call to say hi, her mother would tell me she'd gone to the mall with her sister or to the Inner Harbor with her dad or to the movies with her brother. Against all odds, she was doing great.

She came home at the end of January, about three times faster than the Hopkins staff initially thought she would. She was weak, but all her tests showed everything was in the acceptable range.

But a few weeks later, while at Hopkins for some routine tests, Melissa's breathing became labored. A blood gas test showed her oxygen level was extremely low, and she was admitted to the hospital. Three days later her level was so low she had a tube put down her throat and was put on 100 percent oxygen.

Doctors explained to her worried parents, Shirley and Bob, that the first round of chemo drugs had damaged her lungs and she was now in respiratory distress. She also had a common pneumonia that most people's immune systems could fight off, but because hers had to be destroyed during the transplant, she was losing the battle. Antibiotics poured into her veins but probably couldn't do enough.

Two days later the doctors again delivered bad news to Melissa's folks.

"The doctor who was in charge came in and said they had tried everything, but she wasn't responding and there wasn't anything else they could do," Shirley recalled.

"What chance does she have?" Shirley asked, now accustomed to the declining percentages.

"About zero," the doctor said without flinching. "We don't think she's going to make it."

"A social worker came in and tried to help us deal with the [impending] death," Shirley said, reading notes from a little green spiral notebook that she kept during the ordeal. "Bob was sobbing."

But Shirley, a no-nonsense kindergarten teacher, listened politely and then swung into action. She called their pastor, who immediately drove the forty miles to Baltimore to pray with them.

"As the day went along and she was getting worse and worse, I asked the pastor if the church elders could come down and pray for her," Shirley recalled.

Within a few hours, a half dozen men joined Melissa's family, and surrounding her hospital bed, they pleaded with God for her life. They sang hymns, including "It Is Well with My Soul," the last song Melissa's sweet soprano voice had sung as a solo at church before her diagnosis. They quoted her favorite Bible verse, John 3:16: "For God so loved the world that he gave his one and only Son, that whoever believes in him shall not perish but have eternal life" (NIV).

"It wasn't real emotional," Shirley recalled. "There were no tears, although [her younger brother] Steve was having trouble talking.

"He was all choked up and kept saying that if she didn't make it, she was going to heaven," Shirley remembered.

Shirley, however, continued to believe that God could heal Melissa.

It was a Wednesday evening, so Bob called their church in Hanover, Pennsylvania, and asked the people gathered for prayer meeting to pray for his dying daughter. He called relatives and friends, including me, as he fought against the odds.

I was devastated when I got the call from him.

"They don't think she's going to make it through the night," he told me, choking back the tears. "Will you start praying?"

I assured him I would, dropping to my knees as I hung up the receiver. I joined Melissa's many friends and family members as we sought God's healing power. Next, I called Marc and Elizabeth and secured their prayers as well.

After the elders finished praying and singing at Melissa's bedside, they left quietly. Melissa was in a coma and totally unaware of what had transpired, including the serene feeling that everyone present said they felt. Just then another doctor came in.

"There's one more thing we want to try for Melissa," the

doctor said. "We don't know if it could do anything, but it won't hurt."

And with that brief explanation, the nurses carefully turned her on her stomach to see if her breathing would improve.

Melissa's mother, who was resting in the apartment across the street, called the nurses every hour to get an update. The report was always the same: "She's holding her own." But in the wee hours of the morning, Melissa's oxygen-saturation level went up ever so slightly.

"When I called the next morning, the nurse said, 'Don't get excited yet, but things are moving up,'" Shirley recalls. "When I heard that I already knew she was healed."

She was right. Against all odds, Melissa made it.

Her family thanked God; everyone who had prayed for her was thrilled. Even the Hopkins cleaning ladies rejoiced!

"Glory, hallelujah," one of them said at the sight of Melissa seated in a chair with the ventilator still in place. "We've never seen a patient intubated and sitting up in a chair."

Exactly one week after the night of prayer, the tube was taken out and Melissa was breathing completely on her own.

"When they took the tube out, the nurses were saying, 'It's a miracle,'" Shirley recalls. "When they discharged her, the doctors were saying, 'It's a miracle.' Of course, the cleaning ladies knew it first!"

Melissa never tires of hearing her mom tell this story because she knows that according to the odds, she shouldn't be here.

"I really feel like I've been given a second chance," she says. "Every time I even go outside and look at a tree, I feel so thankful, because I know I wasn't supposed to be here."

As I write this chapter, Melissa is preparing to start her second year at art school in a couple of weeks. Despite a life-long battle with dyslexia and lingering physical problems caused by all the steroids she had to take following her transplant, Melissa earned all As and Bs her first year. She hopes to become a children's-book illustrator and teach private art lessons. Two months ago she was the maid of honor at her sister Lynn's outdoor wedding, looking radiant with her dark, curly hair and wearing a long, fuchsia gown.

The last four years have caused her to grow up quickly. She has had to deal with losses from the cancer; doctors say the lethal chemo destroyed her ability to have children. It hasn't been an easy road, but there's a trust factor in her life that wasn't there before.

"It's hard to explain, but I feel everything I do now is totally in God's hands," she says. "Once you get to that lowest part in your life, where there's nothing you can do, you learn that He is in control, and you give it all to Him and life is so much better.

"You can't really tell someone that," she admits. "You have to experience it."

Have you learned that life lesson yet? It's one of the most important ones that cancer can teach. But Melissa's right. I can't tell you; you have to experience it firsthand, just like she did and I did.

When I was diagnosed I was told I had, at best, a fifty-fifty chance of surviving. It seemed to me as if someone was going to flip a coin: heads I live, tails I die. It drove me crazy thinking about it.

And then an even better truth hit me: God wasn't playing roulette with cancer.

He didn't have His fingers crossed.
He wasn't going to wish me luck.
He wasn't taking bets on my future.
He didn't need good odds to heal me.

You need to know and believe that cancer is *not* an automatic death sentence. When I heard the word *cancer* in the same sentence with my name, my initial reaction based on the people I knew with cancer was: *I'm a goner.* But that was in

1990, and today I am still very much alive and feel as well as I ever did!

Doctors do their best at predicting cure rates and odds of survival, but these predictions are just educated guesses. I'm very glad Marc does not regularly dole out predictions about how long patients have to live. He feels those predictions become self-fulfilling prophecies in many patients' minds. Every single person in this book lived longer—some *many* times longer—than doctors or medical science would have predicted.

Melissa's mom told me something that helped her deal with the terrible prognosis doctors gave her daughter. When the Hopkins doctor said Melissa had only a 15 percent chance of surviving the bone marrow transplant, he explained that while that statistic was true for transplant patients as a whole, for each individual the chance of survival was either 0 percent or 100 percent. Each one would either live or not live—no in-betweens!

Predictions are just that. They do not have the last word.

When I first thought about writing this book, I didn't think there was any chance my friend Doris (see chapter 11) would still be alive when I got to her chapter. She was already on "borrowed" time. But just last week we spent three hours together, sipping orange spice tea in her sunroom and talking about what I should write about her. I would not be surprised if I get to hand her an autographed copy of this book.

The other day I was visiting in the home of a twenty-three-year-old hospice patient named Jessica. She and her mother had prepared a fabulous lunch of tomatoes stuffed with crab salad, fresh fruit, fresh-squeezed lemonade, and Bavarian apple cheesecake. Jessica has been fighting a rare, incurable adrenal cancer for four years and trusts that God will take her home at just the right time. She told me that a few months ago she overheard the hospice nurses saying she "wouldn't make it through the night."

"It makes me so mad when they say that," she told me, dark eyes fiercely flashing.

I had to suppress a smile. I had never heard a hospice patient complaining about this topic before! Leave it to Jessica to be so mad she refused to die on cue!

"I know I'm dying," she continued matter-of-factly as only Jessica can. "They're trying to prepare my mom and everything, but they don't know when it's going to be—only God does."

Jessica is absolutely right. The Bible makes it very clear: "All the days ordained for me were written in your book before one of them came to be," King David wrote (Psalm 139:16 NIV).

"My times are in your hands," he penned (Psalm 31:15 NIV).

No matter how many (or how few) tomorrows doctors may have told you to expect, those tomorrows are safe with God. We may not know what tomorrow holds, but we know Who holds tomorrow. And that is enough.

Be encouraged: Cancer is not an automatic death sentence. Your times are in God's hands, and He doesn't need "good odds" to heal you.

～ Huberta

"This peace just came over me."

EVERYBODY REACTS DIFFERENTLY to the diagnosis of cancer. Your reaction and mine probably had many things in common, but no doubt there were differences as well. You might have feared cancer for years because other relatives had already been diagnosed. Maybe you checked for lumps and watched for telltale signs, knowing for certain your turn was next. Or you might have thought, like I did, that you had taken such good care of yourself you would *never* have to face such a diagnosis.

But if you were like my friend Huberta, *waiting* to get an official diagnosis was as awful as finally hearing the word *cancer* itself.

Huberta, or "Bird" as her friends called her, came to our office as a new patient in mid-July 1997. She didn't have a formal biopsy but knew she had an inoperable lung mass that was probably cancerous. She needed more tests and the waiting was taking its toll on her.

Her thin frame fidgeted nervously as she sat next to me in the waiting room that first day in our office. Her fingers tapped nonstop on the chair. Her hands shook as she dabbed at her eyes with a crumpled tissue.

Probably so upset she wants a cigarette, I surmised, feeling a surge of compassion for her.

If she's this upset now, what's she going to do if she actually

gets the dreaded news? I wondered, feeling really helpless to
ease her anxiety.

I hate how long it often takes to get medical tests scheduled
and then to get the results. I realize that from an administra-
tive point of view, it usually can't be helped, but I hate it
anyway.

When my family doctor was trying to figure out what was
wrong with me, I had a barium enema test done on a Thursday
and I didn't get the results until Monday. Four days might
sound like good turnaround time to a doctor or a secretary, but
it's an eternity to a would-be cancer patient. I jumped every time
the phone rang and I worried every time it didn't. Now, as a
patient advocate, I try to make sure that if patients are anxious
about test results, they get called back as soon as the results are
available and not just when it's convenient to do so.

But Bird needed to see another specialist for her tests and
there wasn't anything I could do to hurry along the process. I
assured her we'd talk again if and when she got an official
diagnosis of cancer. I didn't expect to see her again for a
couple of weeks.

But there she was standing in the waiting room the very
next afternoon. She didn't have an appointment, and I couldn't
think of her name. (I meet anywhere from four to eight new
patients a week, so it sometimes takes me a while to get the
new faces and names embedded in my brain.)

She was crying again, or maybe she hadn't stopped since the
day before. I invited her to come upstairs to my office, partly
for privacy and partly because up there you don't feel like
you're in a doctor's office. People usually begin to feel more
peaceful as soon as they come in. Somehow, though, I thought
it would take more than a change of scenery to calm down this
patient.

She began to talk about her fears of diagnosis and treatment.
Her name finally came to me. She was extremely upset, and I
was prepared to listen without saying much. I wanted her to

know that I understood and I cared. I also wanted her to feel free to share her problems with me.

But quickly she turned the conversation to spiritual matters and began asking questions about Bible teachings. I don't usually get into such weighty topics the first time I talk with a patient or family member. I feel it's important to show the unconditional love of God first. That means no agendas, no tricks, and no ulterior motives. I just try to love people right where they are and hope they will open the door at some point to discuss spiritual issues.

Well, Bird was opening the door, but I was afraid to walk through it.

"I don't know how to get to heaven," she said, cutting straight to the chase. "How do I get there?"

Take it easy, don't overwhelm her with too much and scare her away, I thought.

"Would you like to know what the Bible says?" I replied cautiously. She did, so I shared with her the truth about how she or anyone else could get to heaven.

She wanted more.

I shared the story of how God had changed my life while I was in college.

She wanted more.

I talked in detail about how to have a relationship with God.

She wanted even more. She started telling me about things she had done in her life that she *knew* were sins but that her friends had said were okay because everybody does them.

I told her she was right, that the Bible does call them sins.

She confessed she hadn't been to church for years. She knew there had to be something more in life. My head and heart started conversing:

Ask her if she wants to pray to put her trust in the Lord.

No way, you just met her.

She really wants to.

It's too soon.

When I think back now, I wonder why I even hesitated for a moment. I always pray that God would help me to share Him with patients and caregivers only when they're ready to listen. I don't want to force my way in or try to beat them over the head with my Bible. I always want to proceed slowly and cautiously, following God's lead.

I hadn't "done enough" with Bird! It normally took weeks, months, maybe even years for someone to be this ready to surrender his or her life to God. Then I heard God speaking to me—not in an audible voice but in my mind: "Can't you see *I've* already done enough in her heart? Are you going to ask her to pray or not?"

"Would you like to pray and receive God's gift of eternal life?" I asked her sheepishly.

"Yes!" she said as she dropped to her knees, crying harder than ever and clasping both my hands in hers.

I can't remember a word of that prayer.

I was so awed at how God had showed her His truth.
So humbled that He would allow me the joy of praying
with her.
So thrilled by her decision.
So grateful that she wouldn't be facing her diagnosis
alone.

I'm sure it's not hard to imagine that Bird and I quickly became close friends. When God arranges a first-time meeting like that, you start wondering what He's going to do next!

Two weeks later Bird got the bad news that it *was* inoperable lung cancer. I say "bad news" because it's always better when a surgeon can cut out the cancer. I don't say "bad news" because Bird's situation was hopeless. Anne, one of the chemo nurses in our office, was diagnosed with inoperable lung cancer back in 1995 and is cancer-free today. (Marc gave her a 10 percent chance of a cure when she was diagnosed.)

Bird went through chemo pretty well and got what Marc called a "nice remission"—meaning the tumor shrank by at least 50 percent.

Within a few months a CAT scan confirmed that the remission—not nearly as nice and long as we hoped—was over and the cancer was in Bird's spine. Soon, Bird was unable to walk. I called her a few days before Christmas, knowing she probably needed some cheering up. Holidays can be very depressing when you have cancer. For the first year or two after my diagnosis, I wondered each holiday if it would be my last, wanting each one to be extraspecial in case it was my final one.

When I called Bird, she didn't sound like she needed cheering up at all.

"This was the worst day and the best day of my life," she said happily. "I'm paralyzed from the waist down, I have a catheter in, and I need help with everything, so it should be the worst day of my life," she said, still with a lilt to her raspy voice. "But a whole bunch of my friends stopped over today to visit me and sing carols for me and bring me tons of food. I don't think I've ever felt so loved. It was the best day of my life."

I thanked her for cheering *me* up and hung up the phone.

As the weeks went by, I visited Bird regularly at home. The one thing she worried about most was having peace about dying. She knew she was going to heaven, but she wanted to feel at peace about the whole process. We prayed often, and I assured her that God's perfect peace would come as He promised.

In January, I stopped to see Bird at her little mobile home, where her two daughters took turns staying with her. I noticed right away on that blustery, cold day that Bird looked different. I wondered if she had done something new to her bleached blonde hair or if she'd put on more makeup. Even her worry lines, no doubt left over from an unhappy divorce, seemed fewer. I couldn't put my finger on it, but her face had a glow about it I had never seen.

We chatted a while, and when I could stand the suspense no longer, I asked her, "Why do you look so beautiful today?"

"I'm at peace," she said simply as her doelike brown eyes gazed into mine. "On Sunday night this peace just came over me and settled in and it hasn't left yet.

"It is incredible," she continued. "It is so beautiful, I can't describe it. I never thought I could feel this way!"

I hugged her and cried tears of joy with her and just kept looking at her beautiful, peaceful face.

It's times like those that absolutely convince me God is always true to His Word. It's one thing to hear the apostle Paul speak of "the peace of God, which transcends all understanding." It's quite another thing to see it on the face of a bedridden cancer patient with no medical hope of a cure. I've seen it on countless faces of cancer patients and their caregivers.

It is a peace that makes no sense.
It is a peace that cannot be explained.
It is a peace that goes beyond our human mind.
It is a peace that only God can give.
It is a peace I hope you'll feel today.

I'd like to share with you the rest of the verse where Paul writes about this peace because I believe it shows us clearly how to get it.

> *Do not be anxious about anything, but in everything, by prayer and petition, with thanksgiving, present your requests to God. And the peace of God, which transcends all understanding, will guard your hearts and your minds in Christ Jesus.*   PHILIPPIANS 4:6-7 NIV

We get peace from God when we take our worries to Him in prayer, all the while thanking Him for all our blessings. He replaces our worries with His peace and it is enough to fill our heart and our mind.

Eugene Peterson's contemporary-language version of the Bible, *The Message,* says it this way:

> *Don't fret or worry. Instead of worrying, pray. Let petitions and praises shape your worries into prayers, letting God know your concerns. Before you know it, a sense of God's wholeness, everything coming together for good, will come and settle you down. It's wonderful what happens when Christ displaces worry at the center of your life.*

This kind of peace isn't just the absence of striving; it's the presence of something much more. Jesus described it for His worried disciples just before His death:

> *I've told you all this so that trusting me, you will be unshakable and assured, deeply at peace. In this godless world you will continue to experience difficulties. But take heart! I've conquered the world.* JOHN 16:33 *The Message*

If Jesus couldn't promise His faithful disciples they wouldn't experience difficulties, I certainly can't promise you anything different. You and I *will* experience difficulties in this world— sometimes including cancer. But I promise you—more importantly, Jesus the Messiah promises you—we can face these difficulties with unshakable assurance, remaining deeply at peace.

I used to think that if only I knew for sure that my chemotherapy was going to work and that it was all right not to get the radiation and that the surgery really got it all, then I could be at peace. If only I had some guarantees that everything would work. I wanted to hear that the chemo regimen I was getting had a money-back guarantee, not a 20 percent chance of working on me. It was so hard to make decisions and face an uncertain future without any guarantees. Even when I got to my five-year survivor mark, I wanted to be guaranteed of a cure and assured that the cancer would not come back.

I didn't get either of these things.

I was so disappointed when Marc, in his irritatingly honest manner, explained to me during my five-year checkup that while the chance of a recurrence had greatly diminished, there was no guarantee I was cured and I should be monitored for cancer for the rest of my life.

I've stopped looking for guarantees here on this earth.

King David had the right idea: "Some trust in chariots and some in horses, but we trust in the name of the Lord our God" (Psalm 20:7 NIV).

Some of you are trusting in doctors or medical science or alternative therapies, but despite what you read, they don't have guarantees. They may or may not bring a cure, but they can't bring you a peace that transcends all understanding.

> *The Lord gives strength to his people; the Lord blesses his people with peace.* PSALM 29:11 NIV

> *You will keep in perfect peace him whose mind is steadfast, because he trusts in You.* ISAIAH 26:3 NIV

> *For he himself is our peace.* EPHESIANS 2:14 NIV

Those are God's words, not mine. The Bible calls God *Jehovah Shalom,* God of Peace. His is the only peace that's guaranteed.

Be encouraged: You can trust God to provide His promised peace that transcends understanding—a peace that makes no sense in the midst of your situation.

~Jack

"It was our first prayer together."

JACK BATTLED TWO big "C"s in his life: cocaine and cancer. The first battle made it clear that God really loved Jack and the second one showed that Jack really loved God.

Both cocaine and cancer took Jack by surprise.

He certainly hadn't planned that by the time he was forty-seven he and his wife, Jeannette, would be smoking an ounce of cocaine a day. He hadn't planned to go a week without sleeping while they partied round the clock. He certainly hadn't planned to stand by and watch as cocaine wracked Jeannette's body with seizures. But planned or not, those things happened. They were all part of a parade of surprises marching down his life.

Jack had been somewhat surprised when one of his relatives showed him and Jeannette how to smoke crack for the first time. He was definitely surprised when another relative turned him in to the police for dealing drugs. But he was really surprised when he heard that God could give him a new lease on life.

"We had tried to get clean numerous times ourselves," Jeannette explained. "We had taken trips to rehabilitation places in the Bahamas, Hawaii, and Florida. We even bought a new house to try and make a clean start, but we celebrated the new house by smoking crack."

Finally, when their grandson was born in February 1989,

they decided they needed to be clean for him. They went first to Alcoholics Anonymous meetings and then started a Narcotics Anonymous group.

"That's when we found God," Jack said. As they experienced their newfound relationship with Him, both their lives turned around and the fresh start that had eluded them for so long was finally a reality. They volunteered with a local drug-and-alcohol treatment center, joined a church, and helped raise their grandson.

By the time I met them nearly ten years later in the summer of 1998, they were still clean, they still belonged to a church, and their grandson was a happy preadolescent. But their love for God had grown cold.

On our office's patient-health-history questionnaire we ask this question: "How important to you is your spiritual faith?" More than 85 percent of our patients answer *important, very important,* or *extremely important,* but Jack wrote in the word *moderate* on his. As I read his questionnaire on a July afternoon, I knew this patient was going to need more than lukewarm faith to face this next surprise.

I was preparing to leave the office that day when Marc stopped me and said he had directed Jack and his wife to come over to his office immediately. They had been at the hospital having yet another test trying to determine why Jack had suffered with blood clots for years.

Marc had gotten a verbal report from the radiologist who had read the scans.

"He's riddled with cancer," Marc told me grimly. "He's got adenocarcinoma of unknown primary."

I don't have any formal medical training, but I know it's not a good sign when you can't find out where the cancer started.

"He's been going from doctor to doctor for years, never finding out what's wrong," Marc continued. "He's in really bad shape. I'm going to admit him directly to the hospital. I'll be surprised if he lasts a few days."

I glanced at my watch. I wanted to stay and talk with Jack and Jeannette after Marc did. I knew they would need some encouragement after the devastating news they were about to receive. But by the time the nurse took vital signs and Marc consulted with them, I knew at least another hour would go by. I was already late for my promised arrival home so I could take my youngest daughter shopping for some things she needed before we left on vacation the next day. We had postponed the trip from the day before when I didn't make it home on time. I couldn't let her down again.

"I'll stay long enough to meet them, but I have to go," I told Marc.

"That's fine," he said. "I just wanted you to know."

I only had a few minutes to get ready for them, but I offered up a quick prayer.

"God, you know I wish I could stay and be with this couple after they hear the news, but I can't. You can meet their deepest need, and You can provide for them emotionally and spiritually whether I'm here or not. It's not me they need to get them through this but You. Please show Yourself to them and let them feel Your presence."

I grabbed a new-patient packet and went out to meet them in the waiting room.

Jack was a big guy, more than six feet tall and almost 250 pounds. He had fair skin; deep blue eyes; and the most beautiful, shoulder-length, wavy gray hair I'd ever seen on a man. Jeannette was short, with olive skin; long, wavy, dark hair; and dark eyes. She looked to be in her mid-forties.

I did a brief introduction, gave them a brochure about "Turning Your Worries over to God" and tried not to think about the fear in their eyes. I took them back to the nurse and apologized for having to leave before the doctor was ready to meet them, which probably wouldn't be for another forty-five minutes, because he still had another appointment before them. As I walked to the front of the office to tell the secretary

I was leaving, Reverend Scott Sager, the hospice chaplain and a local pastor, motioned to me.

"Is that the Chronisters you just took back there?" he asked.

"Yes," I said. "Do you know them?"

"They belong to my church, but I hardly ever see them and I wasn't sure I recognized them," he explained.

> **Now, I know some people might say that was a coincidence.**
> **That Jack's pastor just happened to be there at the exact same time he was.**
> **That he just happened to be there on the exact day when Jack was going to get really bad news.**
> **That he just happened to be there at the exact moment when I had to leave.**
> **Some might say it was a coincidence.**
> **I prefer to call it an answer to prayer.**

I quickly informed Scott about the news Jack and Jeannette would receive. He agreed to remain after the hospice meeting to see them.

Here's how Jeannette recalled that day.

"We came out of Dr. Hirsh's office, and our heads were spinning. It was all so awful," she recalled. "I looked into the waiting room and there was Pastor Scott. I started to cry. I couldn't believe he was there for us."

Scott prayed with the frightened couple and went with them to the hospital while Jack got checked in. He stayed in close contact with them all that next week while I was on vacation.

By the time I returned to the office, Jack had had his first round of chemo in the hospital and was feeling its full effect. I talked with him and Jeannette in Marc's office as they waited for him to come in. We barely knew each other, but already they were baring their souls.

"I'm afraid to sleep at night," Jack said, looking down at the floor.

"Afraid you won't wake up?" I asked, knowing his answer would be yes. I had felt the same way those first days after diagnosis as I awaited surgery. I had known it was illogical, but that hadn't mattered. When I would close my eyes, I would feel a suffocating darkness come over me and would be afraid to sleep because I might not wake up. I had felt silly trying to explain it to anyone, so I hadn't bothered. Thankfully, it had passed quickly.

I asked Jack what, if anything, he did when the night fear gripped him.

"Last night I prayed," he said.

"We even did something we'd never done before," Jeannette added. "We've been together twenty-six years, but for the first time in our relationship we prayed together. When he was so afraid, I didn't know what to do so I held his hand and I prayed out loud for him—it was our first prayer together. Ever since I saw Pastor Scott here in this office I knew God was answering our prayers."

God kept on answering all sorts of prayers for Jack and Jeannette. He answered their prayer for more time, and instead of living a few days as Marc had feared, Jack lived another five months. They prayed for one more vacation and God gave them a glorious few days at their favorite beach, where they just *happened* to bump into a former coworker who handed them a $100 bill for "dinner on him."

"We never felt so close to each other and to God as we did since we found out Jack had cancer," Jeannette told me. "I think Jack grew more in his relationship with the Lord the last five months than he did in his whole life."

At his funeral, Jeannette gave a beautiful eulogy sharing that through his cancer battle, Jack "found a closeness to God that he lacked" and "his faith took on a whole new meaning."

She called his cancer diagnosis a "wake-up call" to get them back on track spiritually. The diagnosis had taken them, but not God, by surprise. God proved that to them (and to me) when He placed their pastor right where they needed him when they needed him. He continued to orchestrate their steps throughout the next few months because they trusted that He was in control and could take care of their needs.

I don't know if your or your loved one's cancer diagnosis has taken you by surprise, but I guarantee it has not taken God by surprise.

He is all-knowing.
He is all-seeing.
He is all-powerful.
He is in control of everything.
He knows what you need and when you need it.

I don't know if cancer is the first or the last in a series of battles you've faced. I talk to many heartbroken people in my office for whom it isn't even the biggest battle they face; it's just the latest blow life has dealt them. It's tough either way.

For me, cancer was the first really difficult battle I'd ever faced. I was unprepared to fight such a formidable foe. Others have faced so many foes that they feel they don't have what it takes to fight one more. Either way, cancer can send us reeling and feeling out of control.

Most of us would have to admit that we like to be in control. I know I do. I like to make plans, carry them out, and then smile smugly at how well they all went. I like to call the shots. I'd rather *tell* God what I need than have Him tell me.

Jeannette expressed it beautifully to me one time when I was visiting the couple and it seemed apparent that Jack was not going to get an earthly physical healing.

"It's really hard to pray for God's will because I know it may not be the same as mine," she said quietly. "But that's really what it boils down to, isn't it? Do I want God's will or mine for Jack?"

She had hit upon the million-dollar question: *Whom do I want to be in control of my life?* Cancer is a wake-up call for all of us. Will we insist on being in control of our life, our future? Or will we relinquish control to the One whom the Bible says has our times in His hand (Psalm 31:15)?

When you believe in God, I think it's hard to come to terms with the fact that He has allowed adversity to come into your life or your loved one's life. David Biebel talks about this fact in his book *If God Is So Good, Why Do I Hurt So Bad?* He says there are two truths suffering people have to reconcile: Sometimes life is agony, and our loving God is in control.[1]

Think about it.
If God knows everything, the cancer diagnosis did not surprise Him.
If God sees everything, He saw the bad news coming.
If God has power over everything, He could have stopped it.
But He didn't.

He didn't stop you or your loved one from getting cancer. He didn't stop it from happening to me, or to Jack, or to anybody else in this book. I don't think His Word promises He will stop all bad things from happening to us. On the contrary, I think it promises that He is prepared for each battle and will equip us.

The Message paraphrases 2 Corinthians 4:8-9 this way: "We've been surrounded and battered by troubles, but we're not demoralized; we're not sure what to do, but we know that God knows what to do; we've been spiritually terrorized, but God hasn't left our side; we've been thrown down, but we haven't broken."

He is in control.
Errant cancer cells aren't.
Toxic medicine isn't.
White-coated doctors aren't.
Herbs and vitamins aren't.

You aren't.
I'm not.

The sooner we learn this truth, the easier our cancer fight will be. It's actually quite freeing once you get it right. You can relax knowing Someone else is in charge—Someone much more intelligent, vigilant, and powerful than you or I could ever hope to be. Psalm 121:4 tells us God neither slumbers nor sleeps. Matthew 10:29-30 promises us that God knows when a sparrow falls and how many hairs are on your head. (Of course, they might be pretty easy to count if you've recently lost them from treatment!)

It's a lesson I keep learning over and over again each day as I walk with the Lord. I learned it again the day Jack died (after he had lived thirty times longer than the doctor's earlier grim prognosis!).

I wanted to be with Jeannette at the end because I didn't want her to be alone. The hospice nurse had left and another would come in a few hours. We thought Jack would go any minute, but he didn't, and the time came that I had to leave because I had to lead the Cancer Prayer Support Group meeting. Just as I had done when I first met this couple, I prayed that God would meet their deepest needs. Jack was already resting quietly in a coma, but I knew Jeannette needed God's strength.

I left their little home, where Jack's hospital bed was set up in the living room. A few minutes later, Jack's son, daughter, and sister just *happened* to stop by. Then a friend came over. She *happened* to get out of work early and *happened* to think of Jack. She also *happens* to be a nurse. She sat with Jeannette, helping her to make sure Jack was physically as comfortable as possible. She was there holding Jeannette's hand when Jack peacefully breathed his last.

Nobody thought it was a coincidence.

Be encouraged: This cancer diagnosis has not taken God by surprise; He is in control and knows what you need.

A Cup of Cold Water

BEFORE I BEGIN Tina's story, I'd like to remind you it *is* a true story. I say that because if I didn't know her and I saw her story on a television movie, I'd say it was pretty unrealistic.

But there's one thing I keep learning in my journey of faith: God doesn't always do things in an easily explainable fashion. Sometimes He does things that can't be measured in a science lab or examined under a microscope. Sometimes He does things that defy natural laws. This story is about one of those times.

It all started innocently enough—with a cup of cold water in our doctor's office, actually. Back in the spring of 1994, before I worked for Marc, I stopped by his office on my lunch hour to visit someone from the Cancer Prayer Support Group who was getting chemo that day. I was right on time for her appointment and planned to see her for a few moments, pray with her, and then leave. But when I arrived I was disappointed to find out that of all days, Marc was running ahead of schedule and she already had gone into an examining room to talk with him before her treatment.

I wasn't too happy about this turn of events. This was supposed to be a quick visit so I could get back to my "real work" in public relations at the local chamber of commerce. Now what should I do? I had promised the friend I'd be there, so I felt I needed to make good on my word. I plopped down in a maroon waiting-room chair and picked up a dog-eared magazine. Pretty soon a conversation with myself began in my head.

Just leave, one voice said. *You said you'd come and you did.*

But I didn't get to see her, the other voice protested.

Just leave a note, the first voice countered. *It's good enough.*

But I told her I'd see her, came the reply.

Just then two women came in the door, interrupting my thoughts. I tried not to stare, but I couldn't help noticing that the younger one wasn't feeling well. She was still dressed in flannel pajamas and slippers. *Probably too weak to get dressed,* I thought to myself, recalling days during my treatments when my goal was to be dressed by noon.

As I watched the careful attention the older woman gave the younger one, I surmised she must be the patient's mother. I looked away and started flipping through my magazine.

My previous two-way conversation continued in my head, and more than once I was ready to get up and leave. But something, or Someone, seemed not to want me to go. I glanced up at the two women again, and as I did, an overwhelming urge came over me to pray for the one who was sick. Now, I am not an impulsive person at all, but I desperately wanted to go right over to her, put my hands on her head, and pray out loud for her.

I can't do that, I thought, deliberately pushing myself further down into the cushioned seat. *What would Marc think if he walked out here and saw me "accosting" a total stranger and praying over her? What would she think if I were so forward?* I decided I shouldn't do it but wasn't sure if it was more *wouldn't* than *shouldn't.*

A thought ran through my head: *She might die.*

She doesn't look that *sick. She's probably just nauseated from a treatment,* the other voice replied.

It came again: *She might die. Are you going to pray for her or not?*

Now I was really sweating. I had to pray for her. I couldn't stop myself. I was still too afraid to go over to her, even though she sat only a few feet away. So I inconspicuously stretched out my right hand toward her underneath my magazine and with my eyes wide open began earnestly interceding for her—for her health and her life. I can't recall the exact words, but I remember my prayer began something like this:

> *Father God, I'm praying for this hurting woman.*
> *I don't know her name or anything about her.*
> *But You know everything about her, and You love her.*
> *Please, don't let her die without knowing You and loving*
>   *You.*
> *I'm asking You to heal her and to reveal Yourself to her.*

I continued to pray fervently, all the while wondering if this young woman really might die or if I just had an overactive imagination. After a few moments I heard the sick woman say to the other one, "It's so hot in here, and I'm so thirsty. I wish they had a water fountain."

Before I had time to think, I stopped my praying and spoke to her. "I know where cups and water are. Could I bring you some?"

"Why, yes," she said, giving me the first smile I'd seen on her face since her arrival.

I quickly darted to the back chemo room, where the nurses knew me from many previous visits. I grabbed a cup and filled it with cold water. My hands were shaking as I carried it back to the young woman—I was so excited to be able to do something to alleviate even a tiny bit of her pain. She accepted the cup with another smile and I noticed what beautiful, big, brown eyes she had—even without any makeup.

Within moments, the door to the exam room opened and the friend for whom I'd been waiting so long came out. She was so glad I had waited. We chatted a while, prayed briefly, and I went back to work. I thought I would never see the sick young woman with the beautiful, big eyes again, but I still wondered why I had felt such an intense urge to pray for her.

It wasn't long before I found out.

A few days later, the Friday of Memorial Day weekend to be exact, Marc called me at home.

"I'm getting ready to go out of town to a retreat all weekend," he explained. "I've got this young woman in the hospital who's not doing well at all. She's thirty-eight and has breast cancer, but I don't know exactly what's wrong with her now. She's got bilateral pulmonary infiltrates, pleural effusions, and an abnormal liver-function test. I'm giving her standard antibiotics, but nothing's working. I don't know if she's going to make it and I think she could really use some support.

"I don't know if she knows the Lord or not," Marc added. "But she told me about this amazing thing that happened to her in the hospital. Do you think you could go over and talk to her sometime soon? I asked her if it would be okay for you to come and she agreed."

"I'd be glad to see her," I told him, happy that he had thought to ask me, although I wasn't too sure what all the medical terms meant.

It sounded so ominous I decided I better get there as soon as possible. We didn't have plans that evening, so I drove over to the hospital after supper, praying on the way.

I don't know what I expected to see as I walked into that fourth-floor private room, but I definitely did not expect what I *did* see.

There, looking up at me from the hospital bed, were those beautiful, big eyes! She recognized me, too, pulling herself up in bed and very excitedly announcing, "I know you; you're the lady with the cup of cold water!"

"I know you," I just as excitedly responded. "You're the one in Dr. Hirsh's office who was so sick."

The words started tumbling out as fast as I could speak.

"I wanted to come over and pray with you, but I was afraid and so I just prayed for you," I said.

I related to her my irresistible urge to pray for her, even blurting out that I was afraid she was going to die.

"I almost did die," she told me.

I pulled up a chair close to her bed, eager to hear this amazing story.

She told me how Marc had come to see her on Wednesday and had told her frankly that her case had him really stumped. He had tried all sorts of things to break her fever and fight the infection that obviously had taken a hold of her lungs, but nothing worked and he was very concerned. They had talked for a few moments about this dilemma and then he had left, closing the door behind him.

That's when she first saw it, she told me.

"I looked at my door and saw the profile of a person," Tina said. "Slowly the person turned toward me, and I knew it was a vision of Jesus. As He faced me, He closed His eyes and slowly nodded His head forward.

"I don't know why I knew, but I knew He was telling me I was going to be okay."

A moment later, she said, Marc had returned to the room.

"He told me he was going to call in the infectious-disease specialist for a consult," Tina recalled.

"I remember thinking that the Lord must have given him that idea," Tina said.

The specialist had come and gone later that day, making some changes in the drugs Tina was receiving, she said.

The vision, meanwhile, remained on the door.

Later that night Tina said she was still feeling miserable and was fighting a high fever. As she gazed at the door, she was afraid she was hallucinating.

"The door seemed like a movie screen. It was like it came to life," she said. The whole scene of the Last Supper: Jesus with His disciples, washing their feet, breaking bread, drinking the wine, flashed before her eyes. She later described it to one of her sisters, who had a strong religious faith. Her sister told her that her description coincided with the biblical account of the Last Supper, even though Tina said she wasn't familiar with it at the time.

Then the scene switched to Good Friday.

"They were nailing Jesus to the cross, and I saw the thorny crown on His head," she said.

"I remember thinking He was showing me that He suffered for us," she said. "I was sitting there just frozen as I watched. My mouth was just hanging open. I couldn't believe God would take the time to show me all that. Afterwards, I thought it was weird that no one bothered me at all during that time. It was like I was supposed to see it uninterrupted."

Then as easily at it had started, the "movie screen" stopped rolling and the vision returned as a lone figure guarding the door, she said.

Marc came back and checked on Tina on Memorial Day. The chest X ray of the lungs showed the pneumonia was gone. Both lungs were clear, and he discharged her that day.

Five years later as we reminisced about that weekend, Tina still recalled Marc's amazement at her unexplainable turn-around.

"He couldn't believe how good I looked and that I was well enough to go home," she said. "The whole thing was like a miracle! No, not *like* a miracle—it *was* a miracle!"

I don't know about you, but I've never had a vision like that, nothing even close. I've never had a remarkable recovery from an unidentifiable sickness, either. But I know plenty of people who have had amazing visions and amazing recoveries, and I believe in an amazing God who can accomplish both.

Anytime He wants.
Anywhere He wants.
Any way He wants.

Notice how I add "He wants"? That's because, while God is a God of miracles, I don't believe we tell God when and where and how He should respond to our needs.

We don't call the shots.
We don't insist on our way.
We don't demand miracles.
We don't name them.
We don't claim them.

God is sovereign. His ways are not our ways, and His thoughts are not our thoughts. Sometimes our prayers are answered exactly as we had hoped—sometimes even better than we had dreamed. But other times He doesn't do it our way.

People often say that God doesn't change, that He's the "same yesterday and today and forever" (Hebrews 13:8 NIV). I wholeheartedly agree—His *character* doesn't change. But His ways sometimes do.

Just flip through the Bible and you'll see that sometimes He intervenes with a miracle; sometimes He doesn't.

The apostles Paul and Silas were miraculously released from prison (the story is in the Bible in Acts 16), but during a later imprisonment Paul was not released and eventually was even beheaded in Rome.

Don't forget what happened to John the Baptist, who preached that the Messiah was coming. He didn't get a miracle release; he was beheaded in prison.

When the early Church's deacon Stephen was seized and imprisoned, he never received a miracle "get-out-of-jail-free" card. Instead, he was stoned to death. (He *did,* however, have a miraculous vision of Jesus and heaven as he was dying.)

God *is* the same.
The same God of love.
The same God of mercy.

The same God of justice.
The same God of holiness.
The same God who can do things as differently in our life
as He wants.

He cannot act contrary to His character, but He doesn't have to act in accordance with our plans or in the same way in each of our lives.

I know there are God-fearing, Bible-believing, Spirit-filled people who will tell you differently. My goal is not to argue with them but to encourage you with the fact that our infinite God is not limited by our finite brains. We cannot add it all up, figure it all out, or completely understand Him. He is too awesome for that.

I remember someone telling me in college, "If God was small enough for our minds, He wouldn't be big enough for our needs." That, to me, is a very comforting thought.

I feel I must be honest with you and tell you that three years after her miraculous physical healing and amazing vision in May 1994, Tina suffered a recurrence of her breast cancer and has been in and out of remissions ever since. Why didn't God take the cancer completely away? I don't know. Why did He give her a miracle of healing then and not now? I don't know. But I do know that Tina is not the same person she was before that memorable week in May.

At the time of her vision in 1994, Tina had some knowledge about God, but she didn't really know Him in a personal way.

"I believed in God, but I didn't really pray much or read the Bible or go to church," she explained. "My [spiritual] beliefs were not that strong."

Tina's whole spiritual life has been changed because of those miracles. She began praying more, reading the Bible, attending worship, and seeking God's will for her life.

One of those prayers was that God would send her a husband, and in the summer of 1996 she married Bryan, the man of her dreams. He, along with her faith, has been her rock throughout her cancer recurrences.

"I can't even imagine going through all this without my husband," she says.

And she certainly can't imagine facing cancer without God's strength.

I don't know exactly what God wants to do in your life or in the life of your loved one . . . and neither do you.

I hope you will pray for a miracle.
I hope you will believe for a miracle.
I hope and pray and believe you may *get* a miracle.

But most of all, I know that you can count on the Creator of the universe to love you with an everlasting love. You can count on the God of all comfort never to leave you or forsake you. You can count on the Prince of Peace to take away all fear.

That's right. The King of kings and Lord of lords will do that for you.

Sounds pretty miraculous to me.

Be encouraged: God is still in the miracle business today.

~Alice

"You're my best friend."

IF YOU'VE EVER seen the old television show *The Beverly Hillbillies* and you remember that spunky character Granny Clampett, you have a pretty good mental picture of my friend Alice.

Remember how Granny always had her own stubborn way of doing things? Her ways were peculiar and surprised all the traditional folks, but they always worked out very well in the end. That's the way my friend Alice was too. She was about the size of her TV counterpart and her long, salt-and-pepper hair was pulled back in a tight bun. Her weathered skin spoke of years of hard work in the sun, and her blue eyes still danced mischievously despite the fact that she was nearing eighty. Once you'd met her, you never could forget her.

Her home was on a road I traveled nearly every day. Even before we met I had often looked at that ramshackle two-story farmhouse and wondered who in the world lived in such a sad-looking place. The paint on the house was long gone and the dilapidated barn next to it was leaning so badly I always figured it would topple as my minivan sped by. The lot was overgrown with weeds and dotted with junk, including an old house trailer. I later learned that the house had no central heat, and Alice and her husband warmed themselves by a kerosene heater.

Once in a while I'd see her outside chopping wood or whacking weeds and I would wonder who that tiny lady was, swinging such a big ax. I could never have imagined that someday she would call me her best friend.

In the spring of 1995, Alice's world met mine.

She came to the Cancer Prayer Support Group meeting with her daughter Louise. In true Granny Clampett style, Alice didn't particularly like or trust strangers, and she firmly announced during our informal introductions that she didn't know why she had come to the group and she wasn't going to talk. Her arms were crossed squarely across her chest.

Seeing the determined look on her face, I wasn't about to argue with her. I figured she was there because God wanted her there, and she would talk when she was good and ready. I gently asked a couple of questions, and I soon discovered that she had "my" kind of cancer—colon—although hers was more advanced, having already spread to her liver.

But for all her tough exterior, Alice was a softy at heart. It wasn't long before we all warmed up to each other and she began to talk.

Alice could always get our group members smiling and laughing. She was the oldest person in our small group, so we all looked up to her like a favorite grandmother. In many meetings, she did most of the talking and we were glad she did. As we swapped stories about the side effects of chemo-therapy and radiation, group members often talked about nontraditional therapies they were trying—things like shark cartilage, herbal teas, or garlic pills. So no one batted an eye when Alice suggested some of her home remedies:

Soak walnuts in whiskey for a few days to relieve diarrhea.

Nibble on a little bit of peach pit for heartburn. "I know they have laetrile in them and it's poisonous, but it doesn't hurt me," she said, looking none the worse for her odd medici-nal habits.

For respiratory problems, she swore by a mixture of honey,

lemon, whiskey, and linseed oil. "If there's somethin' down there in your chest, that'll bring it up," she told us, and her daughter recalled that it had seemed to work on her as a child.

We also discovered Alice had traveled around the world with her older daughter, Mary, and we delighted at pictures of her atop elephants' backs and camels' humps in faraway places. She once confided in me that if things had been different and she had finished high school and could have managed to go to college, she would have studied geography.

Alice and I developed a special bond because we had the same kind of cancer. She felt I understood her because our medical experiences were so much the same.

Not much else about our lives was the same. She told me what I already could surmise: that she had had a hard life. She said relatives, churchgoers, and the community had generally rejected her. She told me someone had tried to burn down their house to get them out of the neighborhood. Her husband, a master violin maker, lost his prized instruments and tools in that fire. Her only son was mentally retarded and lived in a special group home. Her younger daughter had been born with a crippling birth defect and was later further injured in a car accident. Alice's husband, embittered by his own hard life, often made her life even more miserable.

She responded by rejecting most folks and God, as well.

But she remembered having felt "a great love for God" when she was only three years old. She couldn't exactly explain it, but she knew she wanted to know Him and be known by Him. When she grew up, she took her own three children to church faithfully until they were teenagers.

But then something happened in her church that made Alice feel she wasn't good enough and didn't fit in. It might have been her old-fashioned clothes. Or her run-down house. Or her distrust of strangers. Whatever the reason, Alice felt she was not welcome. So she stopped going to church altogether.

When she came to our support group, which meets in a

church building, it was the first time in decades she had set foot in such a place.

Cancer has a funny way of putting everybody on equal ground. It doesn't matter if you're rich or poor, college-educated or a high school dropout, living in a mansion or in a shack. Everybody is "good enough" to get cancer.

As time went on, our friendship grew. Alice lived so close to my home, I gave her rides to our biweekly support-group meetings. Occasionally on a Sunday morning, I'd see her sitting in our congregation, smiling at me.

In the spring of 1996 I asked her to be my guest at our church's Mother-Daughter Banquet, since my mom lives in another state and couldn't make it.

When I arrived at her house to pick her up, she was waiting in her Toyota truck out front like she always did. I had told her she didn't have to do that—that I would come up to the door for her—but she insisted. I figured she didn't want me to come inside, so I respected that. I also figured that when I arrived she'd be dressed in her usual heavy pants, flannel shirt, and work boots, and that was just fine with me.

But there she was looking like I'd never seen her. Her hair was obviously freshly washed and piled in a soft bun on the back of her head. She wore a bright pink skirt-and-sweater set, accented by a matching jewelry ensemble. I detected a light perfume fragrance. She was smiling when she saw me.

"Wow! Do you look beautiful," I told her. She was beaming now. She handed me a crocheted white bookmark in the shape of a cross that she had purchased from a friend. I thanked her and told her it would go right into my Bible, where I would see it every day and think of her. We didn't say it, but we both knew that without a miracle this would be her last Mother's Day.

It's hard to describe the pride I felt at having Alice as my guest at the banquet that night—I was truly honored that she would be my "mom" for a night. We talked, laughed, and then cheered when she won a prize for being the oldest mother there. I knew the evening was tiring her out, but I hated for it to end.

When I called her the next day, she told me she had slept soundly and peacefully that night, better than she had in months.

Another good thing cancer does is help you focus on the important things in life—things like: *Is there life after death and where will it be?* Alice and I talked often about such weighty matters. She told me she had tried to live a good life and if she had been good enough she figured she would go to heaven, and if not, well, she wouldn't. It was as simple as that.

I asked her if she wanted to know what the Bible says about getting to heaven and she said yes. I shared with her Ephesians 2:8-9: "For by grace you have been saved through faith; and that not of yourselves, it is the gift of God; not as a result of works, that no one should boast" (NASB).

I explained to her that the Bible says nobody is *good enough* to get to heaven, but *anyone* can get there by turning from sin, believing Jesus died on the cross to forgive our sins, and accepting His free gift of eternal life.

Alice soon came to realize that she could have the assurance of heaven, not because of what she had done for God, but because of what He had done for her.

Shortly after that conversation, Alice told me of a night when she couldn't sleep because of pain.

As she lay on the couch downstairs, too weak to climb the steps to her bedroom, she heard a Voice say to her, "Lift up your hand to God." So she stretched out her skinny, little arm and lifted her hand, palm up, toward the heavens in an act of surrendering her physical and emotional pain to God. Her eyes filled with tears as she related the story. She told me that the pain had left her body as mysteriously as the Voice had come and that a sweet, peaceful sleep had then come over her.

I can't explain why God answered that prayer and only took away Alice's pain that night and not every sleepless night. But I am confident that on that night, the God of the universe heard the prayer of a woman who had little by the world's standards, letting her know that He loved her just the way she was.

The last time I had any lengthy conversation with Alice was on a Sunday afternoon in October 1996. We read the Psalms together, and she told me she was ready to go home to God.

"I love God," she kept repeating to me, even though she barely had the strength to speak.

"He loves you, too," I promised her, grateful that she had found her way back to Him.

I can't remember the first time Alice said it to me, only the amazed, grateful feeling the words stirred in my heart when she told me, "You're my best friend." I knew she really meant it. Alice was a straight shooter. She didn't say things to flatter people. It was a humbling moment for me.

Alice's best friend.

Why, I had so many friends there weren't enough hours in the day to be with them all. So many close friends, I would hate to have to choose a "best friend." I had done so little for and with Alice that I felt embarrassed by her pronouncement. I certainly hadn't done enough to earn the coveted designation of best friend. It was so undeserved, so unconditional . . . just like the Father's love for all of us.

I resisted the temptation to protest.

Instead, I thanked her and hugged her frail little body close to mine.

I told her I loved her and she would be my forever friend.

Do you, like Alice, ever feel you're not good enough for God? Maybe you even feel you weren't good enough and that's *why* you got cancer. In the first couple of days after my cancer diagnosis, the devil brought to my mind all kinds of sins I had committed and good deeds I had omitted.

I felt alone.
Worthless.

Condemned.
Defeated.
Not good enough.

At one point I was so low I told my husband, "I guess God really doesn't love me." I don't remember saying that and even now I can hardly believe I was that despondent, but I was.

I even believed I wasn't "good enough" to be physically healed by God. Oh, I never doubted He *could* heal me, I just didn't think He would want to.

"Everyone prayed for Ralph's first wife, and she still died," an evil voice whispered in my ear. "You don't think you're better than she was, do you? If she wasn't good enough to be healed, you certainly aren't."

Thankfully, my dear friend Sheila stopped by during this time and explained to me that my fight with cancer was a spiritual battle as well as a physical battle, and I needed to be reminded of Ephesians 6:16: "In every battle you will need faith as your shield to stop the fiery arrows aimed at you by Satan" (NLT). Those "fiery arrows" often include depression, loneliness, fear, anxiety, and despair—all common emotions for people facing a life-threatening illness.

Sheila prayed with me and reminded me what I knew in my head but could not feel in my heart: God's love and presence in our life are not based on whether we're "good enough"— they are gifts, unconditional and with no strings attached.

Slowly but surely, I began to feel God's love again and to understand that my prayer for healing would not be answered as a reward for good behavior.

So I remind you today, you *don't* have cancer because you weren't good enough. And you *don't* need to do something special to earn or deserve healing from God. Don't try to bargain with Him by being an especially good person, hoping He will reach down and heal the cancer. I've seen Him heal people who didn't even thank Him afterward, and I've also seen really "good" people who didn't get healed here on earth.

The way God feels about you is like the way Alice felt about me: He considers Himself your best friend. There's nothing you can do to make God love you any more—or any less— than He already does. He proved that a long time ago:

"This is real love. It is not that we loved God, but that he loved us and sent his Son as a sacrifice to take away our sins" (1 John 4:10 NLT).

Be encouraged: Cancer is not a punishment for bad behavior, nor is healing a reward for good conduct. God's love for you has no strings attached.

The Other "Cancer"

I DON'T KNOW how long you've had cancer or how many cancer diagnoses you may have had—I know people who have survived three or four different cancers—but this is a story about a man with two cancers.

One of them he had for fifteen years, and the other "cancer" he had for more than forty years. One was in his body, and the other was eating away at his soul.

God didn't cure one, but He did miraculously heal the other.

One cancer made this man think he didn't need anybody else's help, the other made him realize how much he really did.

Both cancers showed me once again that blessing can come when God and cancer meet.

I would never have met Lyle if not for the fact that I just *happened* to be on the second floor of the hospital that day in November 1997 and I just *happened* to see a nurse who knew me and who just *happened* to have spoken to Lyle's family doctor about me.

"Lyle is in his seventies and was diagnosed with leukemia about fifteen years ago, but he's in the final stages now," the nurse told me. "The doctor just told him to go home and get his affairs in order, and I think the doctor wanted you to talk to him about getting ready to die."

Great, I sarcastically thought to myself. *I'm sure a dying man is going to want to talk to me, a perfect stranger, about such a personal subject.*

I felt very inadequate for such a task, as well as reluctant to be intruding on such a private time in someone's life. But pushing those feelings aside, I said a quick prayer for wisdom and walked down to the private room number the nurse had given me.

Lyle was in the bed and it was obvious to me, even without any medical training, that he was very physically ill. He looked thin, pale, and fatigued as he lay on the hospital bed, propped against some pillows. What wasn't obvious to me was that he was harboring an emotional pain that was also taking its toll.

His family doctor was in the room and introduced me as someone who might be able to help him "get things ready to die." They discussed a possible hospice consult, and then the doctor left us alone.

It was an awkward moment. When someone is near the end of life, I consider it a rare privilege to be allowed to share those personal times and I wasn't sure this dear gentleman really wanted me there. He said he wasn't really feeling well, so I suggested I come back tomorrow when we could talk more. He agreed and I said a short prayer with him before I left. My first feeling was one of relief.

Even though I'm a definite people person, I'm also very aware that not everybody else is and I don't want to be perceived as pushing my way into a sick person's life and making him or her feel worse. (Like the well-meaning stranger who showed up on my doorstep a few days after I came home from my surgery and proceeded to explain to me that if I only had taken *her* brand of vitamin supplements I wouldn't have gotten cancer.)

As I turned the corner out of Lyle's room and headed through the door and down the stairs, a feeling came over me that I can only describe as one of expectancy.

I know many people who often have feelings about things, but I'm not that way. Even though I'm an empathetic and caring person, my head tends to lead the way most of the time. So when a feeling like this comes over me, I know it's from God.

I didn't have any logical reason, but I sensed He wanted to do something really special in Lyle's life. I hurried down the stairs, praying for Lyle and believing that he was going to experience what I call a "divine appointment"—one of those meetings that God arranges at just the right time and place so He can show His power in someone's life.

When I got back to the office I excitedly told Marc about the "chance" meeting and my feelings that God wanted to work in this man's life. Later that day I shared the story with my husband and with Marc's wife, Elizabeth, asking them both to begin praying for Lyle. It's been a real blessing to have Elizabeth as my prayer partner for several years (our husbands also pray together regularly). We meet weekly and she joins me in asking for God's special touch in patients' lives.

The next day I hurried over to the hospital at the appointed time, but Lyle said he still wasn't feeling too well. I left a devotional booklet for people who are ill and prayed with him and his wife. I felt disappointed and wondered if maybe he was making excuses not to have to see me. I came back to his room a few days later and got a similar reception.

Maybe I should just leave this poor guy alone, I thought as I left after just a few moments with him. Still, I couldn't shake the notion that God had something special in store for him. So I continued praying and asking others to do the same.

It was now thirteen days since my original introduction to Lyle. I knew his longtime chronic lymphocytic leukemia had gone into the final acute stage and he had very little time left. I decided to try one more hospital visit.

This time Lyle seemed to want to talk. He told me his neighbor just *happened* to mention to him that he knew me and that I would be a good person to talk to. I began to sense immediately that I was not intruding and he really hadn't been feeling well enough to talk during my other visits. Lyle asked my advice about what he should do when he went home.

I certainly am neither a professional counselor nor a social worker, but I've walked with enough people down this road to have learned some things.

I asked him what practical steps he already had taken in preparation for his imminent departure from this life. He carefully outlined steps he had taken with his will, his funeral arrangements, and information his wife would need to know after he was gone. Every time I suggested something he should do, he already had done it. I could easily see he was an incredibly kind and caring person. He wanted to make sure that his children had remembrances from him and that his wife would have clear instructions about her upcoming areas of responsibility.

I could think of nothing to add to his methodical list. He was even using this time to say good-bye to friends and family and to make sure important things were not left unsaid.

"There's a sense that your diagnosis is a gift," I told him gently. "Many people die without warning, but you've been given a chance to get ready and to make things right before you go."

He agreed and said he had been trying to look at it that way. Then I asked him a question that I often ask dying cancer patients: "How do you feel about being spiritually ready to die?"

At first I thought he had misunderstood my question when he began to talk in a hushed tone about an incident that had happened more than forty years ago, but I soon realized that he was unburdening the other "cancer" that had been eating away at his soul.

He proceeded to tell me about an incident that had happened in the 1950s, when he was a board member in a church in another state. There was a matter concerning the pastor, which Lyle, then in his thirties, had spoken up about during a meeting because no one else had the guts to say what was on their minds. His comments were made out of concern for the pastor's well-being, he said. But the pastor took things the wrong way and the next Sunday when Lyle came through the reception line after the worship service, the pastor wouldn't shake his hand or speak to him.

Things continued that way for a couple more months, and Lyle kept feeling more hurt each week. Finally, he couldn't take the rejection anymore and he left the church. That story isn't such a surprising one and, sadly, is played out in congregations around the country each week.

But it was what happened next, or rather didn't happen, that was weighing down this dying man.

Lyle *never* became part of another church again. Oh, he and his wife often talked about the fact that they *should* go to church, but the pain they had experienced in that other church was so strong, they didn't want to risk ever being hurt that badly again. So they went on with their lives, never giving up on their faith in God but also never worshiping Him with others or sharing their gifts with fellow believers in a congregation.

"I cannot tell you how sad I feel that I have stayed out of a church for so long," Lyle told me as a tear trickled down his wrinkled cheek. "I still know God, but it's been so long, I'm afraid He doesn't know me.

"I'm afraid I might not get to heaven because I've been away so long," he said as his voice choked with emotion. "I haven't even talked with anyone about all this for over twenty years."

I can't even remember all I said to my new friend, but there was no doubt in my mind that this was the moment of expectancy I had sensed and prayed about for almost two weeks.

I asked if I could sit down by him on the bed, and the words just began to flow out of me. I asked him how he thought people get to heaven and he accurately explained that we need to place our faith and trust in Jesus and what He did for us on the cross and then live like we believe it. I knew he had done both those things, but there was this one matter that he needed to get straight with God. I had no doubt that God would forgive him. I just hoped Lyle could forgive himself.

We talked about God's unconditional love and His amazing grace and that it was never too late to come back to Him. We talked about Lyle forgiving himself and letting God forgive him too for his unfaithfulness to the church during these four decades. The tears were streaming down Lyle's face by then. We talked about the story of the Prodigal Son and how his father's arms were open and waiting for the wayward boy to return home.

"God is waiting for you, too, Lyle," I told him. "You can't erase the past forty-some years, but you can make sure the remaining time is different."

I prayed with him, probably one of the most emotionally intense prayers I've ever prayed with anyone, as now this broken, dying man was clenching my hands and sobbing like a baby. We prayed for forgiveness for the things he didn't do that he should have done, and we prayed for him to forgive the pastor who hurt him. We prayed about using whatever time he had left to continue to serve God, and we prayed that God would take this whole ordeal and use it for good in Lyle's life.

"That's what I want to do—I want to draw nearer to God," he said when I finished.

I had never seen anyone cry out forty years of guilt and unforgiveness before. I want to tell you that it is an awesome sight to see a person freshly forgiven, released from a prison of his own making, and headed straight into the loving arms of his Creator.

Finally, both our tears began to subside and I left his room.

Later I kept thinking about how Lyle had said he didn't even have a pastor to preach his eulogy. I asked my pastor-husband if he would do it. He agreed, so a few days later I called Lyle's home and spoke with his wife. She appreciated the offer but said it wasn't necessary.

Since I had seen him, Lyle had contacted a pastor friend he knew more than fifty years ago (the gentleman was now in his eighties) and this man had come with his own pastor to visit Lyle. The two had agreed to do Lyle's funeral together when the time came.

Nine days later—many, many years after his initial cancer diagnosis but just one month after our first meeting—Lyle died.

At his funeral, I loved hearing the older pastor talk about how Lyle and he had rekindled their friendship shortly before Lyle's death and how Lyle had drawn close to God in a very special way during his last days.

Most of all I loved knowing I had the precious privilege of seeing God show Lyle that it's never too late to forgive and be forgiven.

One of the phrases Lyle said to me in his hospital room that day of divine appointment keeps echoing in my mind: "I can't believe I left the body of Christ."

He kept saying it over and over, still amazed that he, a "pillar" of the church, had left the family of God and stayed away over half of his life. It was the one big regret in his life.

It reminded me of another cancer patient my husband had ministered to after a mutual doctor-friend introduced them. That man, a very successful businessman with a lovely home and family, said the one thing he regretted was that he had neglected his spiritual life. He, too, had missed out on the joy of worshiping, fellowshipping, and serving with other believers. He spent his last weeks reading Scripture with my husband and trying to make up for lost time in establishing a relationship with God. It was a bittersweet time.

I didn't have any idea I would be writing this book when I met Lyle, but if I had told him about it, I feel confident he would have asked me to implore people not to let anything keep them from finding and being a part of a congregation where they could grow in their faith and help others do the same. Lyle realized, almost too late, that we were not meant to be lone rangers; instead, we were created for community.

Are you a part of the family of God?

I don't mean are you going to heaven. I mean are you a part of His family right now here on earth? Do you have a worship home where the Bible is taught, lives are changed, and those with needs are ministered to? Are there people who pray regularly for you, encourage you with God's Word, and help with any practical needs in your life? If not, you are missing out on one of God's greatest gifts on earth.

I know there are hypocrites in churches and I know there are swindling preachers and everything else rotten you can imagine, but don't let other people's failures keep you from the truth that we were created to live in community.

The apostle Paul explains this truth in 1 Corinthians 12:12, 26: "The body is a unit, though it is made up of many parts; and though all its parts are many, they form one body. So it is with Christ. . . . If one part suffers, every part suffers with it; if one part is honored, every part rejoices with it" (NIV).

We need each other; that's a lesson cancer drives home quickly. One of the saddest things I see is cancer patients who have no "spiritual family" to help them through the tough times. After I was diagnosed with cancer, I remember thinking, *Well, there's one good thing about the timing of this: I can't think of a better church to be in. I know they will take care of my husband and children for me.* And the church did. They brought home-cooked meals (including dessert, which I never gave my family), baby-sat my children, sent cards by the hundreds, and prayed fervently for my healing. I can't imagine going through my cancer battle without them.

If you aren't part of a congregation because you've been hurt in the past—or for any other reason—I pray you won't let anything keep you from finding a worship home. Hebrews 10:25 admonishes us not to "give up meeting together, as some are in the habit of doing" (NIV).

God wants to touch you through His family. He wants you to touch others the same way. Don't miss out for forty years like my friend Lyle did. It was almost too late when he finally saw the truth.

If you are a part of a growing, loving congregation I pray you'll do two things:

1. Allow people to care for you, and
2. Keep giving back in whatever way you can.

Allowing people to care for you can be hard. It's often easier for people to be givers instead of receivers, and cancer puts you in the latter category more than you probably will like.

Within two days of being diagnosed with cancer I already disliked being on the receiving end. People offered to do things for me, and I didn't want to let them, even though I was very physically weak from all the "clean-outs" my body had been through to try and diagnose my problem. One day a fellow churchmember named Sheila set me straight about givers and receivers. She called and offered to come over and clean my bathrooms and put sheets on our guest bed because my parents were coming in from Ohio for my surgery.

"No way," I told her. "I can't let you clean my toilets!"

She kept insisting and I kept arguing. Finally, she put an end to my protests that day and for all the years since with her wisdom: "Don't rob me of the joy of doing this for you."

Ouch! I had never thought of it that way. Sure, it gave me joy to do for others, but I hadn't thought about it giving them joy to do for me!

I set out the toilet-bowl cleaner, the toilet brush, and clean sheets for Sheila.

Giving back to the family of God can be hard when you're going through a health crisis.

My dear friend Judy, who had chemo with me back in 1990 and faced a recurrence six years later, is a faithful member of a large local church. Little by little, she had to cut back on all the ministries she enjoyed in the church. Finally, she wasn't able to do any of the things she had done, so she has found a new ministry.

She sends out the Cradle Roll packets to the parents of newborn babies. Every few weeks she mails another letter of encouragement to new parents. The newsletters are printed already, so all she has to do is address them and mail them at the right time. She can do it lying on the couch dressed in her cozy bathrobe if she needs to. She says it's not much, but I'm sure it means a lot to those new parents.

I'm positive that in God's amazing way, those newsletters often arrive on just the right day to cheer a discouraged mom or a frustrated dad. I'm sure Judy blesses dozens of people without ever leaving her home. She has made sure she remains faithful to her church. A "little thing" like cancer is not going to stop her from giving back.

I wish I had met Lyle when he was well, and I wish he had come to my church. But I didn't and he didn't. He never was well enough to attend another worship service, but I'm so grateful that one day I will meet him again and he will be whole and we will be a part of the same heavenly congregation forever.

Be encouraged: The family of God is a gift from God especially for times like these.

∽ Doris

"It's not the miracle we prayed for."

FOR CANCER PATIENTS and their caregivers, all of life can be divided into two parts: B.C. (Before Cancer) and A.C. (After Cancer).

I knew Doris B.C. In fact, she's the only person in the book whom I've known both before and after cancer.

My last happy B.C. memory of her is November 1996, when a group of us women from church were on our annual all-day Christmas shopping trip to area malls. I actually don't like to shop, especially not on a Saturday with a crowd of people, but I went every year for the good food and fellowship. (I even went while on my chemo treatments, although I remember spending most of the day in restrooms and on benches!)

It was time for our traditional dinner break at a Mexican restaurant conveniently located between two big malls. I was sitting by Doris, who's just a couple of years younger than I am and has three daughters close to my kids' ages. But that afternoon we were acting more like junior-high girls than grown-up mothers.

We all noticed a sour-faced gentleman seated at the table next to ours who seemed very bored. One of the women in our group said she thought she could get him to smile. Karen has a way of always making people laugh. She borrowed a tube of red lipstick with a pocket mirror from Doris and began smearing the bright shade all around her mouth, clearly missing her lips. Then she turned toward the unhappy gentleman, waited to catch his eye, and flashed him a bright red grin. He never cracked a smile, but we were hysterical. I thought Doris was going to hyperventilate from laughing so hard.

Four days later there was nothing to laugh about in Doris's life.

She'd had a seizure while talking on the phone with a close friend. An ambulance took her to the nearest hospital, where brain scans showed a golf-ball-sized tumor near her right ear. A biopsy provided a grim prognosis: It was malignant and a Stage IV glioblastoma multiforme, the most aggressive and deadly kind of brain cancer.

A doctor told her she probably had six months to live.

As I write this chapter, that was three *years* ago. Just last month she went to the beach with her family for a week. Last Sunday she was in the worship service at church, and last week she sipped tea with me on her porch.

That doctor was wrong by a factor of at least six times. That's because neither the doctor (any doctor) nor the patient is in control when it comes to the A.C. Only God knows. And because by faith we know Who knows what lies ahead, we can rest in His love regardless of what predictions are made or what complications arise.

Chances are you won't have to go through anything remotely similar to what Doris has gone through, but I believe you will still be inspired by God's amazing touch in her life. If by chance you do have a difficult road such as Doris's to walk, I believe you'll be encouraged to see how, against all odds, God is carrying her through.

We know she's had a miracle, even if it's not the miracle we prayed for.

Before Doris was diagnosed with cancer, she directed our church's cantatas—elaborate music-and-drama productions that usually fill the local high school's nine-hundred-seat auditorium a couple of nights each Christmas and Easter. She also directed our Vacation Bible School each summer, during which a few hundred children descend on our church grounds for a week of Bible stories, crafts, and games. Doris was, and still is, well known and well loved throughout our church and our community. She didn't have hundreds of people praying for her healing, she had *thousands* of people praying for her healing.

> **They all believed God could perform a miracle of
>   complete healing.**
> **I believed God could perform a miracle of complete
>   healing.**
> **Doris believed God could perform a miracle of complete
>   healing.**

"I remember praying in the hospital when I got the word it was a brain tumor," she said. "I said, 'Lord, I'm not ready to leave this world yet. I want to see my girls walk down the aisle. I want to sit in the front row at three graduations, and I want to hold grandchildren. I need more time.'"

Doctors tried to buy some more time for Doris with daily radiation treatments designed to reach the remaining tentacles of the tumor that had remained untouched by the neurosurgeon's scalpel for fear of risking permanent brain damage.

About halfway through the six-week course, she started having seizures and some impairment in her movements. The deadly tumor was growing. It had only been a couple months since her first brain surgery, but because she had healed so well and there was no other recourse, the surgeon went back in again. Experimental chemotherapy wafers about the size of dimes were placed in the hole where tumor was scraped out. (The wafers slowly erode, releasing concentrated chemotherapy to the tumor.)

Again Doris healed quickly. But by summer, symptoms returned, signaling the tumor's return. In September 1997 she underwent a third surgery even though her prominent neuro-surgeon said he had never done this surgery more than twice on anyone. More chemotherapy wafers, now no longer experimental but officially approved for such use, were placed in the spot. It seemed our prayers might be answered after all as the tumor began to shrink miraculously on each MRI.

But then in December 1997, it spun-off another lesion that doubled in size in just a month. By February I was seriously concerned for Doris and spoke to her radiation oncologist about her.

"She seems worse, and I don't think she has much longer," I told him as we talked in my office.

"That's an accurate assessment," he responded. "She could be well for a little while or she could crash next week. I don't think it will be long."

Doris started stereotactic radiation, a very specialized, ultraprecise way of delivering highly concentrated radiation to the brain. She started oral chemotherapy but stopped it because of terrible side effects.

She also started saying her good-byes. Doris decided it didn't look like she was going to see any more high school graduations (Nicky had a year to go and Katie had two years), or weddings or grandbabies (Angie, the oldest, didn't even have a steady boyfriend). So Doris started making memory boxes for her daughters, then sixteen, seventeen, and twenty-one.

"I put in presents for Katie's and Nicky's graduations and something for them to carry down the aisle at their weddings and a note from me," Doris explained.

"What a great idea," I told Doris. "And if God heals you, you can still hand the memory boxes to the girls yourself on those important days."

We hoped for a miracle, but it was getting harder.

As weeks stretched into months, Doris again started to improve and I knew it was a miracle she hadn't died. I rejoiced to see her smiling face at the Easter cantata and then at Vacation Bible School.

But by August 1998, Doris was having bad headaches and her neurosurgeon decided to operate a fourth time. More chemo wafers were put in. Again, Doris healed amazingly quickly.

The headaches lessened and she got used to a "new normal." We both knew, and her doctors agreed, that it was a miracle she was still alive and functioning so well.

In September 1998 we went with a group of sixty women from our church to a huge Christian conference in Philadelphia. Doris and I roomed together with our prayer partners, Mary and Elizabeth. We had a refreshing two days, knowing full well that when Mary had registered Doris for the conference in the spring, there was no medical hope Doris would be alive when the conference date arrived.

We called it a miracle, simply not the one that we prayed for.

So much happened in the next year, it's hard to fathom. Because this is only a chapter about Doris and not a whole book, here's the condensed version: Doris remained in her unexplainable medical remission, Angie got engaged and married to an old friend and had twin boys born two months premature, and Nicky graduated from high school!

Nearly every prayer Doris had prayed that day in the hospital emergency room was answered in the span of less than a year!

Maybe God wasn't going to completely heal the cancer, but maybe it wasn't going to grow anymore.

We believed God for a miracle and it was getting easier.

Then July 1999 rolled around. Doris was still feeling well, but an MRI showed something suspicious. She underwent an unheard-of fifth brain surgery and doctors found an unheard-of brain tumor outside the brain on her forehead. They couldn't get it all and weren't able to put in more chemo wafers.

And that's where things stand as I write this chapter. Doris again has healed marvelously and is back to rocking her grandsons and picking spearmint leaves for tea from her garden. But she still has cancer.

Last week we talked one day about all she's been through and how it has affected her relationship with the Lord.

"I can't imagine how somebody could go through something like this without God," she told me as we curled up on opposite ends of her porch loveseat.

This comment didn't surprise me because I know Doris is a woman of great faith and persistent prayer. She *loves* to pray for people. She has prayer partners she meets with and prayer groups at her home. On Sunday mornings she often calls my husband early in his church office and reminds him she's praying for him as he prepares to preach. She prays for people whenever she's in the claustrophobic tube for one of her many MRIs. ("Shouldn't I get a free MRI after a dozen?" she recently joked with the technician during her umpteenth such test.)

So I asked her how she deals with the question of her unanswered prayer for complete healing, and her answer forms the basis of my encouraging lesson to you.

"I try to realize that while my prayers about my health aren't being answered, there are other prayers that are being answered," she said. "I try to find God showing up in things every day."

She pointed to a lace tablecloth with freshly washed seashells strewn on it.

"I found all those shells while I was on the beach last month," she explained. "I sat down in the sand and started sifting through it with my fingers, and every time, a really beautiful shell would roll out.

"I reached in my pocket and all I had was a hospital sock with the tread on the bottom, but I took it out and put my special beautiful shells in it," she continued.

"Then I got to thinking that me sifting through that sand

was sort of like God moving things in our life out of the way because He wants something special like those little shells to roll out. Some days it's hard not to dwell on the weight of the sand, but I keep trying to sift through it and see something special from God.

"I try to wake up thankful and go to bed grateful."

Are you looking for God today? Where are you looking for Him? Is it just in prayers related to your health or your loved one's health, or are you watching for Him in other places? Maybe in unexpected places.

Every day Doris prays that God will reveal Himself to her that day—that she will see Him and feel Him in some way. And it happens.

Sometimes it's a friend who stops by and takes her out to eat.

Sometimes it's a note that comes in the mail with an encouraging Bible verse.

Sometimes it's a phone call that ends with a prayer for her.

And sometimes God sends someone to her who needs encouragement.

However it happens, Doris looks for joy amidst the struggle in her life. She is not a Pollyanna; she is not an irrational optimist who insists everything is okay when it's not. She is simply a woman who is certain of God's love for her and His plan for her life, even though she doesn't understand the particulars most of the time. She is positive that the facts she knows about the Lord are true despite the way she feels about life sometimes.

"He is not showing up, maybe, the way you wanted, but He's still there," she told me.

Doris doesn't want to trust in appearances or feelings but in the promise of Scripture where the apostle Paul says:

"For I am convinced that neither death nor life, neither angels nor demons, neither the present nor the future, nor any powers, neither height nor depth, nor anything else in all creation, will be able to separate us from the love of God that is in Christ Jesus our Lord" (Romans 8:38-39 NIV).

Are you convinced that neither chemo nor radiation, neither scans nor surgery, neither good news nor bad news, neither predictions nor unanswered prayers, nor anything else in all the world of cancer, will be able to separate you from the love of God that is yours in Christ Jesus?

I hope and pray that you or your loved one gets a quick, easy, complete healing from cancer—I've seen it happen many times. But if you can only find your joy in quick, easy, complete healing, you're going to miss a lot of God. When you, like Doris, can find joy in the midst of troubles and unanswered prayer, you're going to see and feel God as you never have before.

The apostle Paul experienced that amazing comfort and joy and wrote about it in his second letter to the Corinthians:

"All praise to the God and Father of our Master, Jesus the Messiah! Father of all mercy! God of all healing counsel! He comes alongside us when we go through hard times, and before you know it, he brings us alongside someone else who is going through hard times so that we can be there for that person just as God was there for us" (2 Corinthians 1:3-4 *The Message*).

There are a few pretty shells on top of the sand, but most of the really beautiful ones are underneath. It might take some digging, but God will show you where to find them.

Be encouraged: Nothing about cancer can separate you from God's presence; keep looking for Him in unexpected places.

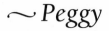

~ Peggy

"God's giving me back
my momma."

CANCER HAS A nasty habit of taking things away from people—
things like hair and strength and jobs and time. Sometimes it
takes them away for a short while and sometimes it takes them
away permanently. Cancer may have already taken something
from you.

**But this is not a story about what cancer takes.
It's about what it can give back.
It's about what it gave back to Peggy.
It's about what it could give back to you.**

Peggy was another one of those patients whom Marc had
bragged about before I worked with him. He never told me
people's names or details about their cancer, just something
about them that really amazed him.

With Peggy, he talked about how amazingly well she toler-
ated the chemotherapy regimen he was giving her. She felt
fine: no nausea, no vomiting, and no loss of appetite. In fact,
her kids often ran out to get her a hamburger or fries to eat
while she was being treated. And if she wasn't eating, she was
smiling. Peggy had a round face; short, curly hair she'd lost a
couple of times from chemo; and a warm smile that endeared
her to children. She had six of her own, four still at home

when I met her, and two unofficially adopted children she'd raised after their own folks had abandoned them.

Peggy told me that her own mother had abandoned her when she was a toddler, and she had rarely seen her in the more than forty years since then. Peggy married at a very young age, was deserted by that husband, and now lived with her common-law husband of many years. She'd been fighting lung cancer for a year and a half when I met her in the summer of 1996.

One day as we chatted in her hospital room she pulled a small, worn photograph from her dresser drawer. She said it was the only picture from her first wedding and she kept it— not because her ex-husband meant anything to her but because of how she looked in the photo.

"That's what I looked like when I was married the first time," she said with a broad smile. "I only weighed a hundred and fifteen pounds. I keep this photo so I can tell my kids, 'See, your momma wasn't always fat.'"

I peered at the little photo. It looked like Peggy's face, but because she now weighed almost three times that much, it was hard to recognize her in the photo.

"You still have the same beautiful smile," I told her, as she flashed a toothless grin for me.

It wasn't hard to see that cancer could not take away much from Peggy—other things had already stolen more than their share.

I had been friends with Peggy for a good six months before I realized she couldn't read. It dawned on me as we talked in her hospital room one day. She hadn't filled out her menu selections for her meals that day, and she asked me to read the choices to her. I had been sending her cards and little encouraging booklets for months, never suspecting that she couldn't read them.

Peggy had a simple faith in God. Because she couldn't read or write, she learned simply by listening. I wasn't the one who shared the Good News of God's love with her; I was just one of the many people God sent to remind her of it.

I know Peggy often frustrated doctors because she didn't follow all their instructions and aggravated secretaries because she didn't remember all her appointments, but she blessed me. Her childlike faith and trust intrigued me because I tend to try and make things complicated.

Probably the single conversation that blessed me most over our two-and-a-half-year friendship happened in May 1997.

Due to breathing problems, Peggy was in the hospital again. (She wasn't in good health when she got cancer, and many of her medical problems were not cancer related.) We chatted for a long time. Peggy was a real people lover and was never at a loss for words. Finally, she got around to the really important thing weighing on her heart.

"You know, there's some good things comin' out of this cancer," she told me in her slightly Southern drawl.

I *didn't* know that, but I was anxious to hear.

"I hate havin' cancer," she continued. "I still wish I didn't have it and that God would take it all away. But I think God's usin' my cancer to give me back my momma."

She proceeded to tell me, without much detail, how her mother, who had abandoned her as a child and whom she hadn't seen for decades, had shown up at her hospital bedside the day before.

"She heard my cancer was back and she came to see me," Peggy said.

She held up a plastic-faced doll wearing a green-and-white crocheted dress.

"She brought me this doll for a present," she continued. "It's the first present she ever gave me in my whole life."

Forty-seven years old and she's never had a gift from her mother. I don't think I've ever seen my mother that she hasn't given me a gift.

Peggy looked adoringly at the doll. I wouldn't have paid

fifty cents for it in a store, but I knew it was priceless to Peggy.

"I think my momma really loves me, don't you?" Peggy finally said.

Forty-seven years old and she's never heard her mother say, "I love you."

"I think your momma loves you a whole lot," I told her. "I love you a whole lot too, Peggy, and God loves you the most of all."

Less than a week later, Peggy showed up in Marc's office with a plastic-faced doll wearing a long, pink-and-white crocheted dress for our staff.

The secretaries thanked her appropriately, but I knew they were baffled about why she wanted to give us such a strange office gift.

I explained to them that the doll was like the one Peggy's mother had given her.

It represented love and hope and forgiveness and a whole lot more.
It represented a healing of something deeper than cancer.
It represented something beautiful cancer gave back.

I don't want to give you the impression that Peggy's battle with cancer was made easy just because she received a present from her mother. It wasn't. She struggled with worries and fears just like most of us.

I remember in particular one urgent phone call I got from her several months after she received the doll. She told me she was really angry because the cancer had recurred again and it wasn't curable.

"When I came home from the doctor I was crying when I came in the door," she explained over the phone. "My little [seven-year-old] boy saw me and said, 'What's the matter, Momma, is your cancer back?'

"I told him yes and he started to cry and I got really angry with God and I went into my room and I screamed, 'I hate you, God! I hate you!' "

She was crying again as she relived the horror of those moments.

Thank goodness I knew what to say because I had heard my author-friend David Biebel talk about a similar situation he had had with a friend who was angry with God over the terrible losses in his life.

"Do you know what God wants to say to you after that, Peggy?" I asked.

"No," came her sheepish reply.

I could tell she expected me to admonish her for her rage.

"He wants to say, 'I love you, Peggy! I love you!'" I told her.

"Do you really think so?" she queried through more tears.

"I know so," I assured her.

I hope my words don't shock you. I certainly don't encourage people to hate God or to be outraged with Him. But I do understand that at times we feel incredibly let down, even betrayed, by Him. He knows those thoughts, so why not be honest and express them? I think David felt let down by God when he penned Psalm 22:1-2:

> *My God, my God! Why have you forsaken me? Why do you remain so distant? Why do you ignore my cries for help? Every day I call to you, my God, but you do not answer. Every night you hear my voice, but I find no relief.* (NLT)

I am shocked when I think of some of the things I told God after I was diagnosed with cancer. But I believe that my honesty with God was a step toward emotional and spiritual healing. As we take all our difficult questions to God, it moves us closer to the only One who truly has all the answers.

Have you been able to be honest, really honest, with God? It sure beats putting on a happy face and pretending you're okay when you're not. It sure beats stuffing all those emotions deep down inside where they will only find some other (unhealthy) way to come out later on. And it sure beats not talking to Him at all.

Psalm 139:1-4 tells us that God knows everything on our mind.

> *O Lord, you have searched me and you know me. You know when I sit and when I rise; you perceive my thoughts from afar. You discern my going out and my lying down; you are familiar with all my ways. Before a word is on my tongue you know it completely, O Lord.* (NIV)

God showed me shortly after I finished my chemo just how powerful His mind-reading ability is.

I remember the incident like it was yesterday, even though it was in May 1991. My family and I went with Marc and his family to their Messianic synagogue about forty-five minutes away in Owings Mill, Maryland. I had finished my chemo three months before, and it was the first time we did anything together socially.

The worship service began with about an hour of lively praise music led by their worship band. I enjoyed it immensely and felt very prepared to hear the morning's message, which I assumed would be next.

But instead a man stood up front and said he had been "given a burden" to pray for people that day. He was visiting a relative in the congregation and had never worshiped there before. I thought this turn of events was a little odd, but I kept listening carefully.

He started talking, and then he continued for what seemed like too long to me. It was bordering on preaching, which was supposed to still be to come. I wondered what Marc and Elizabeth were thinking and whether this kind of stuff usually happened there. (I later learned it had *never* happened before.)

Finally, the gentleman said, "I believe there's someone here today with back problems. I would like them to come forward for prayer."

Someone here with back problems? In a congregation of a hundred and fifty? It would be a miracle if there weren't someone here with back problems!

I have to be honest and say I'm usually skeptical of "faith healers." I'm not skeptical at all about God's ability to heal, just about some of what I see and hear on television. This scene was beginning to remind me of that, and the skeptical newspaper reporter in me was taking over.

I tried to keep focused on praying as all the people with back problems streamed to the front. The gentleman laid hands on and prayed over each one. Some he asked to move around afterward to see if their symptoms were improved.

This could take a while.

And it did. Just when all the back-problem people sat down and I thought the sermon would come, the praying gentleman visitor said he thought there was someone there with an ear problem. It might be an ear infection or a hearing problem or something like that, but there were people there who needed to have prayer, he said.

The small sanctuary was filled with families with young children. *Plenty of ear infections here.*

Parents with babes in arms stepped forward. An elderly man with a cane hobbled to the front.

This could take a long while.

I didn't like feeling cynical during a worship service, especially after I had waited so long for this day to worship with Marc and Elizabeth. I kept forcing myself to pray for the people gathered across the front of the sanctuary. But another conversation kept going on in my head.

Who's he going to call up next? People with headaches? Maybe people who are tired this morning? I'm sorry, Lord, I'm sure he means well, but it's obvious there would be people here with these "afflictions" he's mentioning. If You are really speaking to him, tell him about my eye. Tell him about my eye, Lord.

One of the chemo drugs I took had damaged my tear ducts. This caused both my eyes to "water" because the tears had nowhere to drain. People always thought I was crying when this happened. I had surgery on both eyes and it successfully opened the left duct but not the more severely damaged right duct. I always carried a tissue in my pocket or up my sleeve, ready to dab at my tears. It was a constant, annoying reminder of the cancer, which I wanted to forget. I had prayed for healing before, but nothing had happened.

Tell him about my eye. It was more a dare than a prayer request. I wanted to show that this guy wasn't necessarily hearing from God.

I leaned over to my middle daughter, Bethany, who was eleven at the time, and whispered, "If this guy calls for 'teary eyes' to come up, I'm going!" We both smiled at my little joke and bowed our heads again.

Less than thirty seconds later, the praying visitor said he had another "word from the Lord."

"There's someone here with an eye that weeps," he announced firmly. He reached up his right index finger to his right eye and said it again: "There's someone here with an eye that weeps."

If you've ever felt your heart pounding and about to explode in your chest, you know how I felt at that moment. I lifted my head, glanced at Bethany, and raced to the front. Halfway there I turned to see my husband coming behind me.

By now some of the congregation's leaders had joined the praying visitor up front to help him pray for all the "backs" and "ears" that had come up.

"It's me, it's me!" I excitedly told them. "I'm the one with the eye that weeps!" I quickly explained I was a patient of Marc's and what had happened to my eye.

The congregation's leaders laid hands on me and prayed over me, and I felt the power of God almost knocking me to the ground. When they finished I turned to go to my seat. There were still two hands on my back: they belonged to Marc and Elizabeth.

I hadn't seen them come forward to pray for me, nor had I seen the shocked look on Marc's face when the visitor said someone had an eye that weeps. Marc later told me he knew immediately that those words were meant for me. (He also told me he, too, had been very skeptical up until that point!)

When I turned and saw *my* doctor praying for me, the doctor whose treatment had *made* my eye like this, an incredible healing took place inside me. The anger and the hurt and the confusion I felt with God over my cancer diagnosis were healed that day.

The God of the universe had read my mind—my skeptical, doubting-Thomas thoughts—and showed me His power.

For a long time, I thought the physical healing would come, but it never did, despite much more prayer. My eye was never healed and I still constantly carry a tissue to this day.

I don't know why it wasn't healed, but I do know God has many ways to heal. And if I had to choose between a weeping eye and a weeping heart, I'd choose the watering eye any day.

God healed me that day in the deepest part of me. He healed me so much on the inside that it truly didn't matter to me if He healed me on the outside. I knew beyond a shadow of a doubt that He *did* love me even though He'd allowed cancer to come into my life. I knew He was going to use this awful experience to do something beautiful. You already know the rest of the story.

Often we can't stop cancer from taking things away from us. My friend Peggy was unable to stop the disease's attack on her body. I was unable to stop the chemo from destroying my tear duct.

But God always can give things back to us in spite of cancer. In fact, the cancer is often the vehicle He uses to deliver His blessing.

It was the recurrence of Peggy's cancer, not the healing of it, that brought her mother to her side and reconciled their relationship. For Peggy, that recurrence became a reminder of God's power to heal more than just disease.

I just had to stop for a moment and dab my eye as I type this chapter. Do you know what my watering eye reminds me of now? Not cancer. It reminds me that:

God can read our mind.
God can speak to our heart.
God can heal us any way He wants to.

Physical healings are absolutely wonderful. I will pray for them with cancer patients always. But they are not the *only* way God heals and sometimes not even the *best* way. If my friend Peggy had been given the choice between cancer and her momma, I'm positive she would have chosen her momma. The healing of my spirit was what I needed more than the healing of my eye.

The Bible tells us God is *Jehovah Raphe,* the One who heals. Don't ever doubt it. But don't ever limit Him to just one way to heal.

Be encouraged: God has many ways to heal you.

Miracle Lady, a.k.a. Hospice Dropout

YOU'VE PROBABLY KNOWN a few dropouts in your life—people who have dropped out of high school or the military or community organizations. Ruth is the only person I ever knew who dropped out of a hospice program.

Please don't misunderstand me. She didn't drop out because there was anything wrong with hospice. On the contrary, our local hospice has a well-deserved, excellent reputation, and the care she received was professional and loving.

She dropped out because she had such an amazing touch from God that she just felt too wonderful to stay on as a patient. And even more incredible is that the amazing touch came just when her family had completely given up hope.

I first met Ruth in March 1997, when she came to our office for a consultation. She had been diagnosed with colon cancer the July before at the age of seventy-eight, and follow-up tests now showed it had spread to her liver. It was a situation not considered medically curable, but it was one that chemotherapy might slow and buy Ruth some quality time. The weekly IV treatment she received was considered relatively mild as chemo goes. We've had patients in their eighties and even one ninety-one-year-old complete six months of this therapy with no significant problems.

Ruth's treatment course began at the end of March without

incident. I called her the day after her first dose, and she said she felt fine and had no problems. Each week she came in and reported no difficulties in the previous days. But after the fifth· treatment, it was a different story.

She came into the office with her son, Stuart, feeling weak and nauseated, and was having diarrhea. Marc gave her IV fluids to rehydrate her and expected that she would bounce back quickly as most patients do. When she didn't, he hospitalized her for tests and treatment of her dehydration.

Still no one was overly concerned, and family and doctor alike expected Ruth would be home shortly.

"We weren't expecting anything to reach a crisis level," Stuart told me afterward. He was keeping his older sister, Gail, who was in Texas, informed about their mother's condition, but he didn't feel Gail needed to fly to Pennsylvania.

I visited Ruth at the hospital on May 7, five days after she was admitted. I was shocked at how poorly she was doing. She didn't seem like herself and was listless and not talking much. She had abdominal pain and doctors suspected her bowel wasn't functioning or was obstructed. Her blood chemistry levels were severely imbalanced and showed that her kidneys were impaired.

I could see she was really weak, but she did wake for a few seconds and seemed to know me. I prayed with her and the family at her bedside. We prayed for her healing and her family's peace of mind. Stuart, meanwhile, called his sister and told her she better come home after all if she wanted to be able to talk with their mother.

I went back to see her again the next day, after Marc told me Ruth had really declined overnight and he was not sure she was going to make it. She didn't awaken at all, but her son, his wife, and I held hands around her bed and prayed again for her. The looks on their faces told me they were starting to lose hope.

This sudden downward turn was especially upsetting to

Gail in Texas because she obviously was not going to get to the hospital in time to say good-bye to her mother. A similar situation had happened some fifteen years earlier when her father had died from cancer; that time, there also had been no chance for her to say good-bye.

When I stopped in a couple of days later, Ruth was still comatose and was now curled up in a fetal position. She was breathing with the help of oxygen, and bags of IV fluid were her only source of nutrition.

It definitely seemed as if there was no hope.

Gail arrived May 9 and went straight to the hospital. After spending just a few minutes observing her mother, her years of training and experience as a long-term-care nurse made it clear to her that Ruth was dying.

"She was Cheyne-stoking (stopping breathing for a short while), not responding, and had little urinary output in her Foley catheter," Gail later described to me. "The first time I saw her, I wouldn't have given you two cents that she would survive."

She and Stuart talked together about their mother's rapidly deteriorating condition and then discussed it again with the doctors. Everyone agreed that she was very close to dying, there was nothing else to be done, and the intravenous fluids, which were keeping her alive, were only prolonging the inevitable. So, on Thursday, May 12, the IV was removed and the fluids stopped. They decided to leave the nasal oxygen in place to keep her comfortable as she died.

Marc wrote in his hospital notes that Ruth was having a "progressive downhill course" and that she was "really near terminal" when the IVs were stopped.

Stuart called the funeral director and explained that they soon would need his services.

"I made all the arrangements with the funeral home and expected she would die and they would come and get her in the morning," Stuart says.

Everyone had stopped hoping for recovery and was praying the end would come quickly and painlessly. Medically, there was definitely no hope.

Ruth's children continued their bedside vigil. Stuart and his wife, Pamela, took the night shift and Gail, the daytime hours.

Two days later, on Saturday, May 14, daybreak came as expected, but what happened next was something no one expected.

Ruth opened her eyes. She saw her daughter sitting at her bedside near the window of her private room. And she began to talk to her.

Twelve days in the hospital,
seven days in a coma,
two days without fluids,
and dozens of prayers later,
she simply awoke.

Without warning or explanation, she just woke up and started talking with Gail.

"The first thing I remember her saying is, 'I'm so hungry, I want a bacon, lettuce, and tomato sandwich,'" Gail recalls.

Gail assured her mom she would love to get her a BLT, but maybe she better start on something a little more easily digestible first! Nurses and doctors were summoned, another IV was started with fluids, and Ruth began drinking some juice.

Two days after her miraculous recovery, I stopped by Ruth's private hospital room. Unaware of what had transpired over the weekend, I was expecting her to be comatose but thought I'd visit with the family and pray with them. I'd like to tell you that when I walked into the room and saw a woman sitting up in bed, talking, and eating Jell-O from her hospital tray, I immediately realized God had healed her.

The truth is, I thought for sure I was in the wrong room and I started muttering apologies as I backed out the door! But then

I noticed the family members near the bed—it was definitely Stuart and his wife, Pamela.

They saw the look of shock and disbelief on my face.

"Yes, it's her, it really is," Stuart said, grinning.

Ruth looked over at me, gave me a big smile, and spoke to me by name. It was just what we had prayed for, but I, too, had given up hope it would really happen.

Now we prayed together again—this time thanking God for answering our prayers in spite of us.

When I went back to the office and asked Marc what had happened to Ruth (after chastising him for not telling me she was awake), he said he had no medical explanation for the turn of events. Later I read a dictation he sent to one of Ruth's doctors: "We thought she would probably die in the hospital; however, she made a miraculous recovery after being comatose, and she woke up and started eating and actually left the hospital."

And that's how she became known around our office as "the Miracle Lady."

Ruth stayed in the hospital for another week after she came out of the coma, and she and Gail spent many hours both reminiscing about the past and preparing for the future. Even though she had miraculously awakened from the coma, they knew she still had advanced cancer and both thought her death was still very imminent.

"We talked about the funeral, what she wanted to wear and what jewelry she wanted on, and I wrote that all down for her," Gail says. "She asked me if I thought it would be okay for her to wear her hot pink dress and jacket and I said, 'Sure.'

"We picked out the hymns she wanted and everything for the service was all set."

When she left the hospital in a wheelchair on May 18, Ruth still was very weak and went home under the services of the hospice program. But instead of getting worse, Ruth continued to get better. She started driving her car, gardening her beautiful flowers, mowing her lawn, and going out to eat with friends. And within a few weeks she decided she was just too well to be on hospice.

"I felt guilty being on hospice and not really needing any help," Ruth told me when she came in our office for a recheck appointment. "I mowed my yard before I came in here today. I just had to drop out of hospice."

I told her I had known many people who had lived much longer on hospice than anyone ever expected, some even for years, but I never knew anyone who actually got well enough to "quit" the program. We laughed together about her new claim to fame: Hospice Dropout.

We talked for a while longer that day about her miraculous recovery in the hospital, and her eyes shone with a joy rarely seen in terminal cancer patients. It was obvious she was extremely grateful to God for what He'd done in her life and was anxious to tell others.

"I'm going to share my story at my son's church at their next cancer-support-group meeting," she told me, still grinning.

And that's how Ruth was every time I saw her over the next few months: smiling and talking about her miracle. Stuart said she stayed that way right up until the next spring when, at the age of eighty, she passed away—rather quickly and unexpectedly (on the same day they called hospice to come out and re-enroll her in the program).

I knew God had done an amazing physical miracle for Ruth when she awoke from that coma, but what I didn't know was that was only one part of a bigger miracle.

Shortly after Ruth's death, I saw her son, Stuart, when I spoke at his church's cancer support group. That's when I learned about the other miracles Ruth had experienced.

"I had considered my mother a fairly bitter woman before that [miraculous recovery]," Stuart told me. "She was fairly cynical and in general had a bitterness toward life."

He went on to explain that life had been difficult for his mother. She had been widowed fifteen years earlier when his father had died from lung cancer. She also had had plenty of cancer to deal with in the family before her own diagnosis: her mother, brother, and grandfather all had been diagnosed with colon cancer also; her sister, with breast cancer; another brother, with brain cancer.

Gail remembers that after her father's death, her mother "kind of crawled up inside herself and just pitied herself.

"She was an extremely private person, rather bitter and really lonely."

Stuart agrees that is a fair assessment and admits he was amazed at the transformation that took place after her near-death experience.

"But after that [miraculous recovery], that was all gone," he said. "Afterwards, there was none of that loneliness or bitterness."

Her faith, which had been fairly routine, became vibrant and her relationship with God became very personal. She started reaching out to others and was no longer caught up in herself.

"There was a joy and thankfulness that hadn't been in her life before," Stuart said. "She had a testimony of what God had done for her and she loved to tell it.

"My mother's physical miracle allowed a real emotional miracle and a spiritual miracle to take place," Stuart explained. "She was really a changed person. It was a miracle on every count."

Gail says that last year she had with her mother as a changed woman "was an absolute gift from God.

"We got to talk about and share so many things," she says. "We talked about my father and my brother and my life. We had some wonderful reminiscences. I have to believe God gave it to me.

"There were prayers all over the place for my mother, and I

have to believe it was the prayers coming from everywhere which gave her the miracle."

And that is the story of how my friend Ruth beat cancer. Perhaps you're thinking that she didn't beat cancer because it ultimately took her life, but I would beg to differ with you. I truly believe that beating cancer is about much more than being physically cured, even though I know that's what most people mean when they talk about beating the disease.

Beating cancer is definitely about fighting this unseen enemy in an attempt to be cured, and I would urge you to do that with every breath in your body. But I also would urge you to enlarge your view of what it means to beat cancer.

What if Ruth had survived the cancer but had stayed a bitter, cynical woman or even had become more so because of the cancer? Would we say she beat it?

I believe the real victory Ruth had was that final year of her life when she, still riddled in her body with cancer, triumphed over it in her mind and her spirit. She lived those months as a person who had cancer, but cancer did not have her. She was held in the palm of God's hand, not in the icy grip of a disease.

When I was first diagnosed with cancer, many well-meaning friends told me, "You can beat this!" I know those words were supposed to encourage me, but they didn't. Instead, I thought, *Great! Now if I don't live, it's my fault I didn't beat this!*

I felt such pressure to "do everything right" to make sure I beat cancer. I researched vitamins and herbs and natural healing techniques. I listened to tapes by alternative-medicine doctors promising cures for all. I read stories of miraculous physical recoveries. But nobody said beating cancer could be about more than just a physical cure.

For quite a while, I was "beating" cancer—there was no sign of it in my body—but it was beating me. It was controlling my mind, my attitude, and my relationship with God. It was the first thing I thought about each day and the last thing each night. It was hard to enjoy holidays and special moments because I wondered if they would be my last. My prayer time consisted of nothing other than self-centered pleas for my personal healing.

But God gradually began to enlarge my picture of beating cancer as He spoke to my heart: "Whether you live or die from this is up to Me, but how you live is up to you."

The pressure was off. I would do my part to physically combat this cancer, but I would not judge whether I beat it by whether or not I was cured.

I would beat it no matter what because I would refuse to let it conquer me and control my life.

And by the grace of God I did, and I continue to do so more than a decade later.

Once you have cancer, it can continue to raise its ugly head in your life for a long time.

At checkups.
Before tumor marker tests.
With every bump and lump.
During new aches and pains.

Even if doctors consider you cancer-free, you may still have to keep beating the emotional and spiritual effects of cancer for a long time.

Once you've gotten the bad news of cancer, it's hard not to worry that you're going to get it again. Once your body has "betrayed" you by allowing cancer to invade it, it's difficult to trust it in the future.

But beating cancer is not a one-moment or a one-day, once-and-for-all accomplishment.

Certainly, we beat cancer when we are declared in remission or cured. However, we also beat it moment by moment as we allow God, not cancer, to control our thoughts. We beat it hour by hour as we remember that God's power within us is greater than the cancer. And we beat it day by day as we trust in God's strength and not in cancer's weakness.

The apostle Paul knew how to live in spite of his circumstances. He even wrote from chains in his jail cell, "Not that I speak from want; for I have learned to be content in whatever circumstances I am. I know how to get along with humble means, and I also know how to live in prosperity; in any and every circumstance I have learned the secret of being filled and going hungry, both of having abundance and suffering need. I can do all things through Him who strengthens me" (Philippians 4:11-13 NASB).

Paul beat his circumstances.
Ruth beat cancer.
I beat cancer.
You can beat cancer.

Be encouraged: Anyone can beat cancer, because being victorious is not only about being cured.

~ Nicola

The Horse Lady

I KNEW HER as "The Horse Lady" long before I ever knew her name was Nicola.

And if I was writing a brochure for you about amazing things cancer patients have done while undergoing treatment, the Horse Lady would be my cover photo.

She got her nickname from Marc, who initially had trouble remembering her name, but had no trouble bragging about her exploits to me before I worked in his office. His favorite story was how she loaded up one of her prized thoroughbred horses in her horse trailer, hitched it to her pickup, and drove all the way from Pennsylvania to Oklahoma. After delivering the horse to its new owner, she continued to drive herself to Mexico for a vacation.

"Drove the truck herself with her oxygen tank right beside her on the front seat!" he said with a satisfied smile. "She's amazing!"

Don't let her nickname fool you. Yes, Nicola bred, raised, bought, sold, and showed horses, but they weren't her whole life. In fact, she was probably one of the smartest, most cultured, most well-traveled patients in Marc's practice. She spoke three languages and grew up most of her life in Mexico. Her country home, where she lived with her husband and teenage son, was filled with treasures from her world travels.

She had a beautiful soprano voice and for a time had been a professional singer in Mexico.

Nicola was first diagnosed with breast cancer in 1988 at the age of thirty-eight. By the time I met her in the fall of 1996, the disease had spread to her lungs and Marc was amazed that she was alive and continuing to enjoy life.

The first time I saw her she was in the hospital with pneumonia, a travel version of Scrabble at her bedside so she and her mother could enjoy one of their favorite pastimes. She was feeling pretty rotten but was managing to beat her mother anyway. Now, Scrabble just happens to be my favorite game to play with my own mom, so we had no trouble getting a conversation started on that subject.

After a few more hospital and office visits, our conversations turned from high-counting Scrabble spells to the high stakes involved in a battle with a life-threatening illness. I started praying with her, and she started holding my hand just a little tighter and a little longer at each visit. (I have never told Marc this—I guess my secret is out now—but I even played Scrabble with her while I visited her in the hospital. Her mother went downstairs to the cafeteria to get something to eat and they both insisted that I spell in her mother's absence. I felt uneasy getting paid to sit and play my favorite game—even if just for a few moments—but the smile on her face told me it was the right thing to do.)

About a year after I first met Nicola, she did something with me that no other patient had ever done up until that time: She prayed out loud with me.

I'll never forget the moment. I held her hand, as I always did, and asked her if there was anything special she wanted me to pray, as I always did. But when I finished praying out loud for her, she didn't let go of my hand, as she usually did. Instead, she squeezed tighter and said, "Thank you, God, that Lynn is in my life, and thank you for my parents."

It was another one of those reminders that cancer patients give back to me so much more than I ever could give to them.

In November 1997 Nicola came to another of many cross-roads she faced in her long battle with cancer. The cancer in her lungs had damaged her breathing so much that she had to be placed on a ventilator, a machine that breathes for people who can't breathe on their own. A tracheotomy—a surgical procedure that makes a hole in the trachea to provide an airway for patients who require chronic breathing support—could give her a few more months, according to the pulmonary specialist. Without it, she would have a few days or a couple of weeks.

Her faithful husband, Richard, said he would support whatever decision she made. Not to my surprise, Nicola decided to have the tracheotomy. Why not? She'd driven a horse trailer all the way to Mexico, hadn't she? We all knew she was amazing.

But there was something that Nicola didn't know. She didn't know God was even more amazing.

I knew that while she had seen much of the world and been exposed to all sorts of fine culture that most people only read about, Nicola's home had been largely devoid of spiritual things. She told me she believed in God but didn't go to church because there were too many hypocrites there. For several months she had been reading a Gospel of John I had given her. Although she was well read, she had not studied what I consider to be the very best book of all: the Bible.

So when I went to visit her on the November day when she was scheduled for surgery, my prayer was that Nicola would respond to the most amazing thing I know: God's offer of eternal life.

We had been communicating for the past few days with pad and paper, because the ventilator prevented her from talking, but now she felt too tired even to write. I knew there were definite risks involved with the surgery and no guarantees this wouldn't be our last "conversation."

I decided to stick with yes and no questions to make it easier on both of us.

"Are you afraid of the surgery?" I gingerly asked.

She nodded yes—the first time I'd ever heard this self-sufficient woman admit to fear.

"Are you afraid you might die?" I asked even more quietly.

Again the curly brown head nodded affirmatively.

"Do you feel you're spiritually ready to die?" I asked as I peered into her tear-filled brown eyes.

No, she vehemently shook her head, squeezing my hand tighter in hers.

"Have you ever put your trust in Jesus as your Lord and Savior, asked Him to forgive your sins, and accepted His free gift of salvation?" I asked, keeping one eye on the monitor recording her pulse rate so I could make sure I wasn't upsetting her.

No, she again shook her head.

Just then an alarm went off on one of the scads of machines monitoring all the tubes attached to her. A nurse came and made some adjustments to the machine. Another nurse followed with some new medication and still another came in for another task. Finally, we were able to resume our conversation.

Nicola clasped her palms together in a sign of prayer and looked at me with pleading eyes.

"Do you want me to pray?" I said, wanting to be sure I was reading her gestures correctly.

"Do you want to pray for forgiveness and God's gift of eternal life?" I said, all the while thinking how she couldn't even pray a prayer I could hear.

But I knew that she wasn't praying to me or for me and that God promises us in His Word that He knows our words even before we speak them. So I prayed and my dear friend who could make no sounds prayed too.

I don't know what she said in her heart to God, but I was sure it was truly the most amazing thing she'd ever done.

Nicola survived that surgery and went home to her thirty-acre farm, replete with five horses, two dogs, and six cats, to live out her remaining time. Shortly before that Christmas, Marc, his wife, Elizabeth, and I visited her at her home.

Nicola had for a long time wanted to show off her horses to Marc and Elizabeth, both of whom are animal lovers. I knew she felt especially honored he would make the thirty-minute drive to see her at home.

"Don't let the word get out that I make house calls," he joked with her. We drank spiced tea, ate homemade sugar cookies, and looked at mementos from her years of training and showing horses. Marc even sat down at her piano and played a few melodies for her. When it was time to leave, the three of us gathered around her hospital bed, making a circle around her, and we each prayed for her. Then the Horse Lady did another really amazing thing.

She let go of my hand and put her index finger over her trach tube so she could talk.

"Dear God," she said. "Thank You for all the blessings You brought into my life and for all the love that people have shown me. I know You love me and are working for my good through all these kind people and their kind gestures."

She took a deep breath, trying to force enough air into her lungs to finish.

"And I just want to praise You, God, for all of this."

It's pretty easy to thank God when everything's going well in your life.
When you feel good.
When the test results are encouraging.
When the tumor markers are down.
When a remission looks imminent.
When you have your health.

It's a lot harder to praise Him when things—sometimes most things—are not going well. Before I was diagnosed with cancer, I always enjoyed singing in worship, praising God and thanking Him for all my wonderful blessings. Prayers came easily to my lips, especially prayers of thanksgiving, because I had a lot for which to be thankful. In fact, if you had told me there would come a time in my life when I wouldn't be able to pray, I would have laughed at the suggestion and insisted it could never happen.

But it did.

In those first dark days after diagnosis, I literally couldn't pray. When I would read my Bible and then try to pray, the words simply would not form. Instead, tears rolled down my cheeks, sometimes just a trickle and sometimes turning into heavy sobs. The only thing I felt like I wanted to pray was a desperate cry for healing. What else was there to say?

And then I read a verse in the Bible—one I'm sure I'd read many times before, but it never had seemed that significant:

> *And the Holy Spirit helps us in our distress. For we don't even know what we should pray for, nor how we should pray. But the Holy Spirit prays for us with groanings that cannot be expressed in words. And the Father who knows all hearts knows what the Spirit is saying, for the Spirit pleads for us believers in harmony with God's own will.*
>
> ROMANS 8:26-27 NLT

Two wonderful verses about how to pray when you feel you can't pray. They were right there in the Bible, sandwiched between Paul's discussion of suffering and his explanation of how we can be victorious even in difficult times! (Read the whole chapter and you'll see what I mean.)

It was okay that I felt I couldn't pray. The Holy Spirit would pray for me. He would take my "groans" that were too deep for words right to God Himself. And even better than that, the Spirit would know *what* to pray for me. He would pray accord-

ing to God's will. I love how *The Message* renders Romans
8:26: "If we don't know how or what to pray, it doesn't matter.
He does our praying in and for us, making prayer out of our
wordless sighs, our aching groans."

That's one amazing God! He knows that at the times we
need Him most, we may not be able to express ourselves to
Him, so He has His own Spirit do it for us! After I found
that verse, I would often just sit, my hands on my lap,
palms toward heaven, tears rolling down my cheeks . . .
praying.

I never said a word. I couldn't even form cohesive thoughts
in my mind, but I prayed. I didn't worry what or how to pray. I
simply allowed God's Spirit to take my innermost thoughts,
my deepest fears, to God and pray for me.

In time I was able to pray again myself, but sometimes even
now I still practice the kind of prayer I learned when I had no
other way to pray.

Another amazing thing I learned about prayer during my
cancer ordeal is that God has given us prayers we can pray
when the pain is too deep.

I spent the entire six months of my chemo in the Psalms. I
don't think I opened my Bible up anywhere except to the
middle, where my eyes would fall upon a psalm that expressed
my need to God.

Before then, I had never really been fond of the Psalms
because they were so filled with sorrow and complaints.

"I thought you said they were all a bunch of whiners," my
husband said to me one day as I told him how much the
Psalms were blessing me.

"Well, now I'm a whiner too," I said, smiling.

It was true. For the first thirty-six years of my life I had it
really easy. A wonderful, loving home growing up; a good
education; a great marriage; super children—nothing to whine
about. Life had been so good that I had never needed God the
way I did after I found out I had cancer.

Quite to the contrary, the psalmists had plenty of trouble in their lives, plenty of times they desperately needed God's help. So I read the Psalms. Day and night I read the Psalms as my prayers to God.

> *The Lord is my light and my salvation; whom shall I fear?*
> PSALM 27:1 NASB

> *To you, O Lord, I lift up my soul; in you I trust, O my God.*
> PSALM 25:1-2 NIV

> *God is our refuge and strength, an ever-present help in trouble.*
> PSALM 46:1 NIV

> *Even though I walk through the valley of the shadow of death, I will fear no evil, for you are with me.*
> PSALM 23:4 NIV

I believe that those six months I spent praying the Psalms were as emotionally healing as anything I could have done after my diagnosis. I believe that wherever you are in your cancer journey, the Psalms will encourage you as you pray them.

I hope Nicola's story has encouraged you. I hope you believe it is possible to enjoy life even while going through cancer treatments. I probably could write a whole book just about amazing things cancer patients have done while on chemo.

I know a man who earned his green belt for karate while being treated for lung cancer. I know a woman who went to dance class wearing a belt pump that released a continuous infusion of chemotherapy into her while she danced. I know another man who won a racquetball tournament a couple days after his treatment for widespread colon cancer. None of these people was a star athlete or a famous person. Each was an ordinary person doing an amazing thing.

Even more amazing is our God. Amazing enough to bless Nicola through her cancer experience and amazing enough to bless you through yours. Amazing enough to hear the deepest prayers of our heart.

Be encouraged: You can pray even when you feel you can't.

~ Cecelia

So Much Hurt,
So Little Time

I WOULDN'T BE surprised to hear that your name is on a "prayer chain" or two around this country or that people have told you they are praying for you. A diagnosis of cancer usually compels people to pray . . . or at least to talk about praying.

I know that prior to having cancer, I often had been guilty of telling people I would pray for them but forgetting to do so. I even remember phone calls coming through our church prayer chain, and afterward I would get busy and neglect to pray.

I guess that's why I was a little suspect when people told me they were praying for me. I wanted to say, "Are you really? Are you *really* praying for me? I hope so, because some days I am hanging by the thin threads of those prayers."

Of course, I didn't want to sound ungrateful, so I didn't say that to anyone. Instead, I just smiled and said thank you. But it made me think twice about telling someone I would pray for them. I realize that someone else may be hanging on by my prayers, and now when people ask me to pray for them, I usually do it right on the spot so I *can't* forget.

This is a story about a patient who, strangely enough, didn't want me to pray with her.

In case you haven't noticed by now, I'm a people person. I'm an extrovert, which means people usually energize me, not drain me. It's neat how God had already given me all that

I needed to be a patient advocate, even though I was clueless about what it would take. I'm able to connect with cancer patients and caregivers easily, and it's usually not long before we forge fast friendships.

That's what really bugged me about Cecelia.

It was obvious from the start that she didn't want me to be her friend. She didn't want to be my friend, and she certainly had no intention of "connecting" with me in any way.

I met her at the hospital on my day off, because Marc had mentioned to my husband that he had a patient he was very concerned about and would like me to visit sometime. She had been his family's veterinarian ever since they had moved to Hanover almost ten years before.

Now, Marc is *not* a people person, but he is a dog lover, and I knew he cared a lot about Cecelia because she cared a lot about his beloved dogs. (He calls them "Blabs" because they're part bulldog and part black lab. I call them big, because that's what they are.)

Even though Marc wasn't telling me to run right over to the hospital that day to meet her, I figured it was important to him and I had the time, so I went, anxious to make another friend.

Patients are usually quite pleased when I come to the hospital and meet them. I know I would have loved to meet a cancer survivor while I was still in the hospital after my cancer surgery. It would have been great to have someone with whom I could identify and share and receive encouragement.

Cecelia was not particularly thrilled when I came to the hospital. Marc told me she had been diagnosed with lymphoma eighteen years earlier and had been in and out of remissions since that time. She had refused treatment with this last recurrence and her time appeared to be running out.

She was cordial to me, but she was far from friendly. I'm no psychologist, but it was obvious she had signs of depression: one-word answers, little eye contact, emotionless voice, and teary eyes.

I told her about my job and the brief history of my own

cancer experience. I gave her a booklet on "Finding Hope When Cancer Recurs" and a little devotional called "Someone Cares." I tried to chat, but it was obvious the conversation was not going to go anywhere.

Still, she seemed so sad that I asked her if I could pray with her. People *always* want me to pray with them. Since I've started working with Marc, I've prayed with all kinds of people of all kinds of faiths. I've prayed with Jews and Mormons, Jehovah's Witnesses and Baptists, and even with a Christian Scientist, who told me that even though her religion didn't believe in sickness or doctors, she came to our office to get chemo "just to make sure all the bases were covered."

I've prayed with people who told me I was the first person ever to pray out loud with them, and I've prayed with people who prayed really loud *while* I was praying for them. I even jokingly told Marc one day that I must be a really *bad* "prayer," because people always start crying when I pray with them.

But Cecelia the vet was one of only two people I'd ever met who *wouldn't* let me pray with her.

She got really teary when I asked, shaking her short brown bob vehemently.

"No, I have a block against that," she explained, which really didn't explain much of anything.

"I'll pray for you when I leave," I told her. I figured she probably really wanted the prayers, but somehow didn't think they could or should be heard on her behalf.

About ten days later she came into our office, and I greeted her in the waiting room. Icily cordial again. She still was in no mood for conversation or for my friendship. I gave her a booklet about "Living with Cancer" and left her alone.

She was quite sick, and Marc wasn't very optimistic she would get strong enough for any treatment or that it would help if she did get it. I felt a real urgency to try to break through her discouragement and show her a ray of hope. I scribbled off a note of encouragement and mailed it.

A couple of days later her parents took Cecelia to the emergency room with shortness of breath. I hurried across the street to the ER, where I talked briefly with her parents in the waiting room and then went back to check on her. Patients are usually really thrilled when I come over to the emergency room to see them. They always ask me how I found out so quickly and how I managed to drop everything and come right over in their time of need.

Cecelia wasn't thrilled.

She didn't even crack a smile or mutter a thank-you.

I usually don't talk much in the ER, because patients are often on oxygen or heart monitors and need to stay calm. I simply stand by their side, holding their hand or patting their arm, and I know my presence comforts them more than words.

I didn't try to talk to or touch Cecelia. Her own body language had made it clear before that she didn't want my "comforting" touches.

I asked her if I could pray with her, but again she shook her head no.

I tried a different tactic.

"Would it be all right if I just prayed silently over you?" I asked gently.

She thought for a moment and nodded yes.

I noticed she closed her eyes, which surprised but delighted me because I hoped she was praying along with me.

I closed my eyes too, and I stretched out my hand across her body without touching her. I silently prayed, first for her physical health. Then I prayed something like this:

Lord, there are obviously some big walls separating You and Cecelia. I don't know how they got there or why, but I know You can tear them down. There is so much hurt and so little time. I pray she would allow You to remove these barriers and work in her life to meet her deepest needs.

I was careful not to pray too long because I wasn't sure what her reaction would be.

When I finished, there were no tears, no smiles, no thank-yous, nothing to show that anything special had taken place. I left quickly, wondering if maybe I should just leave the poor lady alone from now on.

Three days later Cecelia's parents brought her to the emergency room at around 9 P.M. Her condition had worsened so much that Marc felt she might not make it, and he shared that concern with his wife, Elizabeth, as he rushed out to the hospital.

She later told me about the conversation.

"He said he thought this probably would be it," Elizabeth recalled. "I was getting the girls (then fifteen and eleven) to bed and we were just ready to pray together.

"I told them, 'We have to pray for our vet, Cecelia. She might die.'

"We got on our knees and we earnestly prayed for more time for her," she said. "We prayed that she wouldn't die without knowing Jesus and His love for her—that God would spare her life that night."

Elizabeth later told me she shared Marc's affection for this special lady who had such compassion on their family pets. She also told me about another side of Cecelia, a side I hadn't seen.

"I never saw any animal she wasn't good with," Elizabeth told me. "She was very knowledgeable, very warm-hearted, soft-spoken, and gentle, but always grinning."

The next morning at work Marc told me Cecelia had nearly died during the night but was doing a little better. I headed over to the intensive care unit the first chance I got that day. I planned to stay only a couple of minutes because I knew she was weak and would tire easily.

She was resting in her room when I walked in. I made some small talk and then took the plunge again.

"Would it be all right if I prayed with you?"

Good thing I was in the hospital, because I almost fainted when she said yes!

I stayed calm, though, and didn't grab her hand. I didn't want to scare her away now that the walls were starting to crack. Finally the long-awaited opportunity was here, but I realized I had no idea what to say. I prayed silently that I would know what to pray out loud, and within moments, God began to put thoughts in my mind and I formed them into words.

I prayed for God to reveal Himself to her and I prayed she would give Him all her hurts and fears. I prayed she would trust Him because He loved her and had proven that love by sending Jesus His Messiah for us all.

Still no appreciative response from her afterward, but we *had* prayed together. I knew my job was to be faithful, to pray, and to let God do the rest.

I went back to see her the next day, but I didn't go in right away because I saw she had a male visitor. I noticed he had a Bible in his hand and was quietly reading some verses to her. I didn't know who he was but was certain God had sent him to help bring down the walls. I stayed outside and prayed silently for the man as he shared his heart, and God's, with her. Soon, I looked up and saw him praying out loud at her bedside. I wondered if he'd asked first or had just "prayed away"!

I asked a nurse who the visitor was and she said he was the pastor of a nearby church, where one of Cecelia's siblings attended. He came out of her room and I knew Cecelia would be too tired for another visitor, so I just stuck my head in the door and said, "I'm just going to say 'hi' and 'bye' because I don't want to wear you out. I'll come back another day when you haven't just had company."

I was certain she would feel gratefully "off the hook" and not have to worry about whether I was going to ask her to pray again.

But she motioned me over to the bed. She looked thin and weak, and she had tubes coming and going everywhere. I again protested that I didn't want to bother her, but she insisted I pull up a chair, sit down, and talk.

Well, at least one of the walls is down!

I couldn't imagine what she would say now that she was the one steering the conversation. I inched my chair closer so she wouldn't have to strain to be heard.

"We've never had a chance to talk," she started. Her eyes were warm and clear. Her mouth was smiling, her voice steady. Here was the "other" person Elizabeth and Marc knew.

I can't believe this is the same person I've been trying to befriend for the past two weeks. She doesn't even look like the same person!

Then Cecelia began her monologue, which I wouldn't have dreamed of interrupting for the world.

She told me that she had been diagnosed with lymphoma in 1979 and had taken treatments off and on, always getting a remission. Then last year she had developed some symptoms that told her the cancer was back. She denied to herself that it was happening, and she didn't go to a doctor. She let herself get really sick—so sick that she lost the will to live.

"I had a complete breakdown emotionally, spiritually, physically, and professionally," she confessed. "But now I've decided I want to live and I want to fight back at this disease."

I instinctively reached for her hand, and she reached for my mine and held it tightly. It was the first time she had visibly responded to anything I'd said or done since we met.

I told her I had been praying for her to want to live again and that Marc and his whole family had been praying for her.

"What would you like for me to pray for you today?" I asked, knowing she wouldn't turn me down.

She thought for a few seconds and then said, "Pray that I can trust God and let Him lead me."

I couldn't think of anything that I wanted more to pray for her!

We held hands, tears running down both our cheeks, and I prayed a blessing over her and a prayer of thankfulness for what God was doing in her life.

Cecelia lived almost twenty years after her initial diagnosis of lymphoma, but she lived only ten days after that special day we shared together. I continued to visit her and pray with her until the end. On the last day of her life, she told Marc, "I'm ready to go." Two days later I walked in Cecelia's memory at the local American Cancer Society's annual Making Strides Against Cancer event. It was exactly one month after I had first met her.

You might think it sad that Cecelia died just when she finally wanted to live again. I think it would have been even sadder if she lived, still wanting to die. And if you believe Jesus' words, as I do, Cecelia *is* very much alive: "I am the resurrection and the life. Those who believe in me, even though they die like everyone else, will live again. They are given eternal life for believing in me and will never perish (John 11:25-26 NLT).

I hope your cancer pit is not nearly as deep as Cecelia's was. I later learned that her pit was deepened through several major crises that had touched people she loved, including mental illness, suicide, divorce, and war. She had made a commitment to the Lord many decades ago, but her love for God had grown colder with each crisis.

By the time I met her, she had literally given up hope of ever getting out of her pit. That's why she didn't want me trying to reach down into the pit either.

But the healing touch of God was deeper than that deep pit.

Cecelia never explained to me the process whereby the walls came down, and I never asked, but it was obvious it had happened. I don't know exactly how or when God did it, but there's no denying He did it. My hunch is that He climbed down in the pit with her, and He poured out His love until it was so much that it lifted her right out of the pit.

He can do it for you, too.
He can pour Himself into your cancer pit and lift you out.
He is only a prayer away.

If I could reach out to you right now and take your hand, I have a Bible verse I would pray for you:

> *I pray that from [God's] glorious, unlimited resources he will give you mighty inner strength through his Holy Spirit. And I pray that Christ will be more and more at home in your hearts as you trust in him. May your roots go down deep into the soil of God's marvelous love. And may you have the power to understand, as all God's people should, how wide, how long, how high, and how deep his love really is. May you experience the love of Christ, though it is so great you will never fully understand it. Then you will be filled with the fullness of life and power that comes from God.* EPHESIANS 3:16-19 NLT

Be encouraged: Cancer can be a very deep pit, but the healing touch of God is deeper still.

"Either way she wins."

You can't "catch" cancer because it isn't contagious, but when it hits one family member, it has its own way of "infecting" all the others. I saw how my cancer diagnosis ate away at my husband. He tried to be brave for me and not show it, but it's hard to hide fear and worry. I think he would have rather been the one with the cancer than the healthy one standing by, feeling powerless to change the situation.

If you are the loved one of someone with cancer, you may feel as if you have cancer too. In a sense, you do. We usually tell new patients at our oncology office, "When one person has cancer, it's as if the whole family has cancer."

I believe sometimes it's harder to be the "well" person than the "sick" person. The patients usually get plenty of attention, and undergoing treatment can help them feel as if they are "doing something" to fight back at this disease. Meanwhile, the patient's loved ones are often under an increased workload physically and heightened stress emotionally. And because cancer is a life-threatening illness, there's the real possibility that those loved ones may be the ones left behind.

A tug-of-war of emotions can develop: trying to stay positive for your loved one who's sick and meanwhile trying to deal with the negative thoughts swirling in your own mind.

That's the situation in which my friend George found

himself after his wife, Molly, was diagnosed with late-stage ovarian cancer. It seemed to him as if there was no way to win that tug-of-war and be at peace with his wife's diagnosis and prognosis.

But George soon found out that things aren't always as they seem. He learned the lesson that songwriter Don Moen wrote about:

> **God will make a way**
> **Where there seems to be no way.**
> **He works in ways we cannot see.**
> **He will make a way for me.**

When I called George and Molly to get permission to share their story, they were thrilled.

"I keep telling the story and I've felt for a long time that I need to share it more, so people can know what God can do," George told me.

"It's still very emotional for me when I relive it; I can hardly get through it," he confessed in a tear-choked voice.

As you will see, George's story about Molly (who is still in complete remission) is one of those out-of-the-ordinary kinds. I certainly can't promise that God will replicate it exactly the same way in your life, but I do promise He can and will reveal Himself to you, in His own way and in His own time, if you seek Him.

George took it really hard when his wife was diagnosed with cancer in the summer of 1998. They had been married eighteen years but friends for many more. They used to go camping together with their first spouses. Years after those marriages ended, they bumped into each other at a restaurant, "cried on each other's shoulders," and eventually fell in love, George said. Now in their late fifties, they were enjoying their three married children and seven grandchildren when a cancer diagnosis interrupted their happy world.

"She's my wife, but she's also my best friend," George said. "We talk about everything—no holds barred."

Because they shared everything in their marriage, it made the diagnosis especially painful.

"My attitude was: Yes, she has cancer, but we have cancer together," George explained. "I figured it was a team effort to try and beat it."

Molly had surgery and the ovarian tumor was pretty well removed. Afterwards she opted for six treatments of chemotherapy to try and kill the remaining cancer and keep it from returning. She handled the first treatment quite well physically and emotionally, just as I see most first-timers do. Her response was like most of theirs: "That wasn't as bad as I thought it would be!"

But for George, it was a different story.

He called me shortly after the second treatment to tell me Molly was feeling fine, but he wasn't.

"My wife's great, but I'm a mess," he said. "Is this normal?"

One thing I admire about George is his honesty. Many men try to stuff their feelings down, but he isn't one of them. He told me he wasn't handling things well emotionally and felt like just about anything could make him cry. He said he was consumed with thinking about all the "what-ifs"—especially the fear of losing his lovely wife.

We talked about how normal it is for one person's cancer to "infect" another family member emotionally and spiritually. I encouraged him not to suppress those emotions (even if they included tears) and to keep taking his worries and questions to the One who holds all the answers.

I believed God could heal his troubled heart, but I never imagined He would do it the way He did.

About two months after our phone conversation, George stopped by the office for some paperwork and said he wanted to tell me about something "really amazing" that had occurred a few days before, while he was spending his morning time in prayer. We walked out to the parking lot together and the words quickly spilled out of him.

"Every day I just stretch out on the couch and talk to God. I don't worry about how long I do—sometimes it might be an hour," George told me.

He went on to explain that this particular day he was telling the Lord about all the things on his heart, all his worries and fears for Molly and how helpless he felt in the face of it all. He said he poured out his heart about how he wanted to know for sure that his wife would live—that she would survive this cancer.

"But after a while, I got to thinking about how I was doing all the talking with God and I wasn't doing any listening, so I stopped my monologue and gave God a turn," George recalled.

He remembered he lay there for quite some time, but nothing happened; he didn't feel like he "heard" anything at all.

"So, I continued throughout the day in a listening mode, waiting for some reply from heaven, but I got only silence," George said.

Later that evening as he sat watching a football game on television, he said, he unmistakably heard a voice, and the words were very clear: "Either way she wins."

"I turned to my wife, who was sitting in a chair next to me, and I thought she was talking about the game, so I asked her, 'What did you say?' But she said she didn't say anything," George told me.

"I was pretty sure it wasn't on the television, but I didn't know where else it could be from," he said. "So I went back to watching the game and then I heard it again: 'Either way she wins.'

"I looked over at my wife again and it was obvious she hadn't spoken," George continued. "It was then I realized Who it must be."

George confessed to me that he was pretty excited to think he was hearing from God but felt clueless as to what the message meant.

"So, I just said to myself, not aloud, *What does that mean?*" he recalled. "And then I heard the voice again: 'If she gets better, she wins, and if she doesn't, she goes home to Me and she wins even more.'"

George told me that at that moment an incredible peace immediately came over his troubled mind as he thought about that answer. But his divine encounter wasn't over yet.

A little while later, he said he heard the voice again: "Either way you win too."

"Again I didn't understand the meaning of the words and wondered about them to myself," he recalled. "Again the explanation came to me: 'If she gets better, you win, and if she goes Home, you know where she is and you still win.'"

Now even more peace flooded his soul, he said.

It was a peace that he never thought was possible.
A peace to end the terrible tug-of-war of emotions.
It was a peace that was real.
And eighteen months later, it still is very real.

Even today when I speak to him on the phone, he chokes up when he recalls the day God answered his prayers.

"I get so emotional I can hardly talk about it," he says almost apologetically.

George's prayer time is still the first part of his life every day, but he says his prayers have changed.

"When I pray now I ask for very little because I think I've already been given much more than I'm entitled to," George says.

I'm glad George doesn't feel the need to ask for as much. I believe he's learning, as the apostle Paul did, to be "content in whatever circumstances" (Philippians 4:11 NASB). But I don't believe he got more than he's entitled to. The answer he got from God that gave him such peace is exactly what Jesus promises for every believer:

These things I have spoken to you, that in Me you may have peace. In the world you have tribulation, but take courage; I have overcome the world. JOHN 16:33 NASB

Jesus promises that when we rest in Him, we can have peace no matter what our situation, *especially* when we are going through difficult times. Jesus has overcome the world by overcoming the power of death in our life. Jesus has already beaten cancer and heart disease and AIDS and every other illness that strikes us on this earth.

Death has been swallowed up in victory. Where, O death, is your victory? Where, O death, is your sting? . . . Thanks be to God! He gives us the victory through our Lord Jesus Christ. 1 CORINTHIANS 15:54-55, 57 NIV

George doesn't know the final outcome of his wife's cancer prognosis, but he knows the final outcome for all believers in the Lord Jesus. You or I don't know the final outcome of our cancer prognosis, or our loved one's cancer prognosis, but we do know the final, permanent, eternal, forever outcome for all those who belong to God.

I am the resurrection and the life. Those who believe in me, even though they die like everyone else, will live again. They are given eternal life for believing in me and will never perish. JOHN 11:25-26 NLT

Either way we win! A win-win situation—a solution where you can't lose no matter what. You hear business people often talk about this scenario. They try to solve a problem by coming up with a solution that benefits everyone. It's the ideal, but it's not always possible.

Unless of course, you belong to God.

If you are a believer in Jesus, you cannot lose your battle

with cancer. Your loved one cannot lose his or her battle with cancer. People talk that way, though. They say things like, "So-and-so lost his fight with cancer." But for believers, it's a lie. We can only win. When a believer dies, it may appear temporarily that death has won, but we all know appearances can be deceiving.

I love this quote from evangelist Dwight L. Moody. Near the end of his life he said, "Someday soon you will read in the newspapers that D. L. Moody is dead. Don't you believe it. I shall be more alive than I have ever been!"

I know how hard it is to have this eternal perspective when you or someone you love is dealing with cancer. We tend to cling to life here because it's all we know and all we can see. But whether we live ten years or a hundred and ten, it's a blink of the eye compared to the eternity we'll spend in heaven.

"That's all well and good," you might say, "but what about those who are left behind when someone dies from cancer? It doesn't feel like a blink of the eye if you're the widowed spouse or the motherless child."

That's a good and fair question. It's one I asked myself many times after I was diagnosed with cancer. I felt completely at peace about my own possibility of dying. I truly felt that I had had more blessings in my thirty-six years of living than many people have in twice that length. God didn't owe me anything, as far as I was concerned.

But I couldn't find a peace about my husband or children being without me. I tried to imagine all kinds of scenarios where they'd be okay, but none of them worked. The emotional tug-of-war in my heart was unrelenting.

Then one day while sitting alone on my bed, I had an experience similar to George's. I didn't hear an audible voice, but the one in my head was very clear.

I had been praying about my daughters and my husband and telling God that He had to let me live because I simply could not feel all right about them without me.

They want me. They need me. They love me and I love them so very much, I told God.

Then I heard the voice in my mind: "I love them even more than you do."

I know You love them, but I want to take care of them.

"I love them even more than you do," was the reply again.

I know You love them, but they need me.

"I love them even more than you do, and until you can entrust them to My care, you will never have peace," was the response.

I started to cry. In my heart of hearts I knew this was the only way, but the emotional tug-of-war had a few more yanks left in it.

I don't want to entrust them to You, Lord. I want them to be entrusted to me. I want to be in control. I . . . I . . . I . . .

But I knew I couldn't have it both ways. So I told God, "I do not see in any way, shape, or form how my children could be fine or even better off without me. Thinking of them without me is a pain too deep for words. I believe the only thing that makes sense is for me to live. I cannot bear the thought of their grief if I die and of not being there to watch them grow up.

"BUT . . . I am choosing to set aside these feelings and believe You and Your Word. I believe that You love them more than I do and that You can care for them with or without me. I believe You are faithful and trustworthy and You have proven Yourself throughout my life and, in fact, throughout all history.

"So, I will quit trying to figure it out, understand it, make sense of it, or control it. I simply surrender my will to Your will. I will walk by faith and not by sight. I believe in You."

I believed that God through Jesus had proved His love for me.

I believed that either way I would win.

I believed that God through Jesus had proved His love for my family.

I believed that either way my family would win.

When I did that, an incredible peace came over me and has not left me even as I write this chapter nine years later. Surrendering our own life to God is a hard thing to do, and I believe releasing our loved ones into His care can sometimes be even harder to do. But it can be done.

George and I both know.

Be encouraged: God loves your loved ones even more than you do.

~ *"Joe"*

"I can't tell you how much better I feel."

I GUESS I should tell you up front that this is a story about a person who, many years after being diagnosed with cancer, was getting ready to die. I hope you won't stop reading because of that. I believe it has a message for you, whether you, too, are preparing to leave this world, or whether you're planning on being around for a long, long time. It's not really a story about dying; it's much more a story about really being alive.

A story about how good God's forgiveness feels.
A story about how powerful God's Word is.
A story about how amazing God's timing is.

Thanks for staying with me on this one. Since you did, I'd like to introduce you to my friend Joe, a patient I met in Marc's office in May 1996. Joe was in his late seventies, and more than ten years had passed since he first was diagnosed with bladder cancer.

He was a short, stocky, grandfatherly-looking guy with kind, green eyes and a warm smile that probably made his grandkids want to crawl up in his lap. He had enjoyed years of remission from cancer, but by the time I met him, he had begun chemotherapy due to a recurrence. Like many of our patients, he was feeling well despite his grim prognosis, and he was still working at his part-time job at a local grocery store.

I'm still amazed at how well patients can look and feel while going through such toxic treatments. Before I had chemo, I had a picture in my mind of how awful it was going to be. But I have to say that for most people it isn't nearly that awful. In fact, that's what nearly all our patients say when they finish treatment: "It wasn't as bad as I thought it was going to be." Very few get sick from their treatments, and most are able to keep up with some sort of a normal (albeit slower) life.

Just the other day I was showing a young woman around the chemo room, because her mother is trying to make a decision about whether to take chemotherapy for her newly diagnosed cancer.

"Why don't they all look sick?" the woman asked me as she gazed around incredulously at the patients relaxing in recliners, sipping freshly brewed coffee, and licking donut frosting off their fingers.

I explained to her that while taking chemo is no picnic, it's usually not as awful as it was in years past or as most people imagine it will be.

Joe was a good case in point. Just to look at him, you wouldn't have thought he had medically incurable cancer. But he did, and several months after I met him, we both knew his time was getting short. He was admitted to the hospital on a Saturday in mid-March with pneumonia.

On Tuesday morning I headed over to the hospital, which is just across the street from Marc's office, to visit his patients. I always pray as I'm walking the short, tree-lined path, asking God to show me who needs a visit and what would encourage each one. I have all the patients' names and room numbers written on a three-by-five card, and I often pray about whom I should visit first. Sometimes I just do my visiting in a logical fashion: I start on the fourth floor and work my way down, or I start on the second and go up.

Other times I start with whom I think is sickest or most in need of encouragement.

But Joe didn't fit any of these categories that day. I had actually started up the steps to another room and felt God telling me (not in audible words but in the gentle prompting in my mind) to go back down and see Joe. It didn't make a lot of sense to me because he hadn't seemed that sick or that discouraged when I had seen him a few days earlier. Besides, I had planned to see Joe later in the afternoon anyway. But instead I heard what the Bible calls the "still, small voice" of God and I went to Joe's room.

He was happy to see me, but we didn't make much small talk. Instead, he cut right to the heart of the matter at hand.

"I'm getting ready to die, and I'm trying to get my affairs in order," he said bluntly as he labored to breathe with the help of plastic oxygen tubes running into his nose.

When sick people tell me they're dying, my first instinct is to say, "No, you're not—you'll be okay; don't give up."

But I've come to realize as I minister to people with medically incurable illnesses that many times people want to talk about their dying and nobody wants to listen. I think people usually know when they are dying, and if we love them, we'll let them talk about what they're thinking and feeling.

I remember one patient I visited in the hospital who told me she knew she was dying. Her husband, who was at her bedside, got a horrified look on his face and turned to me.

"She's not dying. Tell her she's not. Tell her she's not," he begged me, his voice getting louder and more agitated.

I was caught in a terrible dilemma of not wanting to invalidate the patient's feelings and not wanting to upset her husband even more. I mumbled something about "nobody knowing for sure" and changed the subject. *I'll come back tomorrow and talk with the patient alone,* I thought to myself.

She died the next day before I got there, and I knew I had let her down.

I wasn't about to let Joe down. So when he said he was getting ready to die, I didn't argue. I simply pulled my chair closer to his bed and said, "Tell me about it."

He told me he had written his living will and gotten a hospital social worker to witness it. He also had tried to write down all the practical things that his wife would need to know about and take care of once he was gone.

"There's one other thing I've been trying to do," he said.

"What's that?" I asked, curious since it sounded like he already had all the points covered.

"I've been trying to remember all my sins," he said very matter-of-factly. "I hope I haven't forgotten any."

I was rather taken aback at his words. Over seven decades of living and he was trying to remember every wrong word, deed, or thought!

"Wow! That's a lot of remembering," I said, trying to stall until I thought of something more profound to say.

He said he had gotten the idea when he was on vacation in North Carolina recently.

"I knew I should go to confession as soon as I got home, so I did," he said. "I just hope I haven't forgotten anything."

I let his words sink deeply into my mind. As I thought about Joe's words, I realized he was telling me that he wanted to be sure he was ready to meet God. I felt a wave of joy tinged with sadness as I considered this. Encouraged that Joe took sin—anything that displeases God—so seriously and knew he needed forgiveness, and saddened because guilt seemed to be weighing him down even now.

"I've got some good news for you," I finally said, breaking the silence. "Even if you can't remember every single sin, I believe the Bible teaches us you can still be forgiven for every one."

He started to smile and was listening eagerly, so I began to share Scriptures with him that spoke of God's power to forgive sins. I told him that the Bible does say we should admit our sins to God, but we can do that even if we can't exactly recall each one.

I told Joe that I had had a life-changing spiritual experience in college and I had tried to think of everyone in my life (nineteen years at that time) whom I had wronged. I wrote letters or called them confessing my sin and asking for forgiveness. I have no doubt I missed some sins, but I also have no doubt that God forgave them as well because He knew I would have admitted them if I could have remembered them!

God looks at the attitude of our heart as most important (1 Samuel 16:7). I have known people who faithfully went to confession in their church each week but who were not changed by that act; it simply eased their conscience for another seven days.

I could tell Joe wanted more than his conscience soothed. He truly wanted things to be at peace between him and his Maker, and I don't think his concern is that unusual.

A few years ago I read a Gallup poll on spiritual beliefs and the dying process, which showed that 56 percent of the respondents were concerned about not being forgiven by God before they died and 51 percent worried they might be removed or cut off from God while dying.

I knew Joe needed to know what was going to happen to him after he died.

"There's really nothing we can add to what Jesus did on the cross for us—He paid the price for our sins," I finally told him.

"I was just thinking about that the other day too," Joe responded. "I was thinking about what God had given up when He sacrificed His only Son for us and it made me start to cry."

Again I was both saddened and encouraged. Encouraged that Joe would understand the incredible gift God gave us when He sent His Son into the world and saddened that he did not seem to have any assurance that when he died he would be in heaven. So we looked at the Scriptures again and talked of knowing for certain where we'll spend eternity—not because we are perfect but because we have a perfect Savior. We prayed together, reaffirming Joe's trust in Jesus alone to forgive all of his sins and take him to heaven.

A young respiratory therapist in dark green scrubs came into the room and offered Joe a breathing treatment, but Joe said he was feeling so good he didn't think he needed one. The therapist checked his breathing and said he'd stop back a little later.

Joe and I resumed our conversation, but I didn't want to tire him out too much, so I offered to read Scriptures to him while he rested. He leaned back, sometimes closing his eyes but never his ears as he let the peaceful words of God fill his mind.

I love to watch Philippians 4:6-7 in action: "Do not be anxious about anything, but in everything, by prayer and petition, with thanksgiving, present your requests to God. And the peace of God, which transcends all understanding, will guard your hearts and your minds in Christ Jesus" (NIV).

"I can't tell you how much better I feel," Joe said with a big smile after I told him I was going to leave so he could sleep.

"I started to feel better as soon as I saw you come into the room," he said. "And now I feel so good, I feel like I could get up and dance around this room."

I explained to him that when I came into the room, it was the presence of God in me that he felt touching his heart, and as we talked, it was the peace of God coming over him and calming his mind. He clasped my hands in his weathered ones, thanking me profusely and imploring me to come again the next day and read some more of the Bible to him.

I hugged him, amazed at how much better he looked physically, and promised I would be back the next day.

I glanced at my watch as I went down the hall. It was after 11:30 A.M. I had spent so long with Joe that I would have to come back later for the rest of the patients.

Marc was busy in the office when I returned, and I didn't have a chance to tell him about my wonderful time with Joe.

I always like to share exciting conversations about spiritual matters with Marc because if it wasn't for his generosity in paying me to be a patient advocate, I wouldn't have a front-row seat to so many special touches from the Lord. I want Marc, at least vicariously, to share the joy.

The next morning when I came in to work, Marc matter-of-factly told me Joe had died.

"What? That can't be!" I responded. "I saw him yesterday. He was doing well. We had a great conversation."

"He was incoherent when I saw him during my rounds yesterday at about five o'clock," Marc said. "He died a little after four this morning."

Later I read in Marc's summary that Joe was "very weak, lethargic, and unresponsive" when he saw him later that Tuesday.

I couldn't believe it. Less than six hours after he was chatting amicably and ready to dance around the room, Joe was incoherent, and not even twelve hours after that, he was gone. He had looked—and felt—very much alive when I saw him.

So that's what the forgiveness of God feels like for someone.
So that's what the peace of God can do for someone.
So that's what somebody looks like when they know they're going Home.

If God can do that for someone who is in the last moments of life, imagine what He can do for the rest of us any old time!

Think about it. People with medically incurable cancer are not the only ones who are "terminal." Ever since the Garden of Eden, we've all been diagnosed as "terminal." Ever since Adam and Eve disobeyed God and ate of the forbidden fruit of the tree of the knowledge of good and evil, God says we all have to die physically. You and I already had a life-threatening illness long before we got cancer!

Sin is the disease and "terminal" is the diagnosis.

Cancer or not, nobody gets out of this world alive. Even if we receive miraculous or medical healings here on earth, we will eventually die. Ever since Adam and Eve got kicked out of Paradise, we've been sojourners on our way back to our real home. The apostle Peter understood that clearly and describes us as "aliens and strangers in the world" (1 Peter 2:11 NIV).

But sometimes things are going so well here that we forget that. I know I did. We start feeling like this earth is home and we want to live here forever. But when a diagnosis of cancer comes along, it can be a good reminder that all of us—cancer patients or not—are just passing through.

One day when I was bemoaning the fact that life was hard and unfair, my husband correctly pointed out to me that if everything were easy and fair on earth, I wouldn't have the longing for heaven that God wants me to have. He was so right. I was longing for "the good old days" B.C. (Before Cancer), and God wanted me to be longing for Him and the great days to come in my future home with Him.

It's so easy to forget that you and I were created for fellowship with the Father and that any other relationship is second best.

When I got cancer I had to face this question: *Which do I love more—my life on earth or my relationship with God?* It's easy to say we love God most of all, but when push comes to shove (or a cancer diagnosis comes our way), will we be longing for our heavenly home or only hanging on to our earthly one? Don't get me wrong; I don't think God wants us to turn our back on our family or our home with some sort of misdirected heavenly gaze.

He wants us to love our family with an unending, unconditional love.
But He still wants us to love Him more.
He wants us to love life with a passion and a purpose.

But He still wants us to love Him more.
He wants us to love this world with care and concern.
But He still wants us to love Him more.

Longing for heaven doesn't mean we love people or life here any less, it just means we love God even more. I believe this longing is described in Romans 8:22-25:

> *For we know that all creation has been groaning as in the pains of childbirth right up to the present time. And even we Christians, although we have the Holy Spirit within us as a foretaste of future glory, also groan to be released from pain and suffering. We, too, wait anxiously for that day when God will give us our full rights as his children, including the new bodies he has promised us. Now that we are saved, we eagerly look forward to this freedom. For if you already have something, you don't need to hope for it. But if we look forward to something we don't have yet, we must wait patiently and confidently. (NLT)*

A diagnosis of cancer is another one of those groans as we wait for our new, immortal, heavenly body. I confess that I, like most people, want heaven here on earth. I want Revelation 21:4 to come true *now* for all the sick people I know:

> *He will wipe every tear from their eyes. There will be no more death or mourning or crying or pain. (NIV)*

But that's not a promise for now on earth. It's a promise for later in the new heaven, after the first heaven and the first earth pass away. God promises He will one day make everything new! (Revelation 21:5). In the meantime we hope for what we do not have, knowing that one day it will come.

If you or your loved one has cancer, life has not been fair to you. But please remember this life is not all there is. Enjoy the home you have here for however long God leaves you here, but if you are a believer, never forget it's not where you really belong.

I wish you could have seen the joy on Joe's face just a few hours before he died.

You wouldn't be so afraid about going Home.

Be encouraged: Cancer is a good reminder that heaven is our real Home.

~Dr. Marc Hirsh

A Physician Meets the Great Physician

I KNOW THIS book is supposed to be stories from cancer patients, but I have one more encouraging story I want to share with you and it's not exactly from a cancer patient. It's from a cancer patient doctor . . . my doctor, Marc Hirsh.

But it's not just his story; it's more of my story too.

It's the story of how a Jewish physician met the Great Physician, forever changing his life—and mine as well.

Most of all, it's another story of God's amazing intervention in our life.

When I was getting chemotherapy, Christian friends usually were excited that I was being treated by a physician who had strong spiritual faith and often asked me, "How did this little town manage to get a Messianic Jewish oncologist who is so well trained and respected in his field?" I used to reply jokingly that God sent him here just for me.

Now I know there was much more truth to that statement than I could have fathomed at the time.

A diagnosis of cancer, or any life-threatening illness, normally brings with it many emotions. Thankfulness is not usually on the list. When I found out my cells had gone awry and allowed cancer to grow inside me, gratefulness was the *last* thing I felt.

But I kept thinking about the admonition in the Bible to "give thanks in all circumstances" (1 Thessalonians 5:18 NIV). I knew enough to understand that did *not* mean I had to be some sort of masochist and praise God for every awful thing that happened to me. Instead, I believed it meant I could have a thankful heart no matter how depressing my circumstances were.

So a few weeks after my diagnosis, I began to look for something for which to be thankful. It was another one of those conversations between my head and my heart.

Let's see . . . I have cancer at the age of thirty-six after taking good care of myself physically. No, can't think of anything worthy of thanks there.

My three little girls may have to grow up without a mother. Nope, that doesn't work either.

I'm going to have to take toxic chemotherapy, when I don't even like to take an aspirin. Not much there to feel grateful about.

Finally, it came to me.

Dr. Hirsh! I have a Messianic Jewish oncologist—who knows, maybe the world's only Messianic Jewish oncologist—living just seven miles from my home. I humbly bowed my head and heart and for the first time since hearing the dreaded news "you have cancer," I thanked God in the midst of my circumstance.

"Father, you know I don't feel any happiness about my situation, but I want to thank You for leading Dr. Marc Hirsh here to be my doctor."

I can only imagine God smiling and saying, "Now you're getting it. Just wait to see how really thankful you're going to be for him when you see how I am going to use this doctor to change your life."

The path that brought Marc to a personal relationship with God is a far different one than my own spiritual journey. I was raised in a Christian home and came to a deep, personal faith through the ministry of Campus Crusade for Christ while I was a student at Ohio State University in the early seventies.

Marc, meanwhile, was raised in a liberal, Reformed Jewish home in a Jewish neighborhood in the suburbs of New York

City. In addition to his public-school education, he attended Hebrew school two nights a week and Sabbath services in the local synagogue. His family observed the Jewish holidays, and he had his Bar Mitzvah at age thirteen.

He recalls that most of his religious knowledge came from the Siddur prayer book—a collection of Hebrew prayers and writings based on the Old Testament, the Talmud, and other Jewish sages.

"My family rarely read from the Bible, but my parents instilled in me and my brother a strong sense of Jewish identity, culture, and Zionism (the right of Jews to live in and control the land of Israel)," he says. "I was versed in the lessons of the Holocaust and the history of anti-Semitism but had no personal prayer life or relationship with God—basically no interest whatsoever in Christianity."

Marc describes his upbringing as affluent and his mind-set as materialistic. His parents encouraged him from an early age to become a physician, and he willingly pursued that occupation. After graduating from Johns Hopkins University in 1973, he received his M.D. from Albany Medical College and did his residency in internal medicine at what was then known as Baltimore City Hospital.

"At that time in my life, my medical career was going well and I had accomplished everything I had set out to do," he explains. "I felt no need for God or religion, including Judaism. In reality, I doubted God's existence, and my life's philosophy could have been summed up as: 'Eat, drink, and be merry. Enjoy life to the fullest. And do your own thing.'"

In spite of his less-than-stellar personal life, the young doctor's professional life was going very well by the summer of 1979. He was a successful, well-respected, third-year resident.

But Marc, at age twenty-nine, was about to have a divine appointment that would drastically change his personal and professional lives: He met a lifeguard named Elizabeth at his apartment-complex pool.

As he lounged by the pool, drinking beer and taking hospital calls on his pager, he couldn't help but notice something about this attractive lifeguard in the shimmery blue swimsuit: She was often reading a little black book.

"I didn't know she was a Christian, but I did notice a joy and peace in her life that I lacked," he recalls.

A friendship began and they "spent hours discussing and debating the reality of God and the significance of the Bible, both Old and New Covenants," says Marc, who found it both fascinating and ridiculous that this woman believed the answer to his own existential crisis about the meaning of life could be found in those timeworn pages of the little black book.

Eventually this "theological friendship" took another turn and Marc asked Elizabeth for a date.

"I asked her to go to a bar for a drink, but she said she didn't go to bars," he remembers. "So I asked her to go to a disco, but she said she didn't go to discos. Then I asked her to go to the movies, but she said it depended on the movie."

Exasperated but not dissuaded, he blurted out, "How about dinner—you *do* eat, don't you?"

So they finally settled on a dinner, and the friendship and discussions continued.

Eventually, she challenged him with these words: "If you pray and read the Bible with an open mind, God will reveal Himself to you."

He took her up on the challenge and agreed to let her buy him a Bible. ("Make sure it's not one of those 'trick' ones with the words of Jesus in red," he insisted.) And "just to prove her wrong," he started reading right from the first page with Genesis chapter 1.

But a strange thing happened as he read—he began to sense "a Presence" around him.

"The words on the pages began to restore meaning to my life," he recalls. "By the time I finished reading the Old Testament, I had decided God really *did* exist and I wanted to lead a Jewish observant lifestyle.

"I debated whether to read any farther in the Bible because I knew that Jesus was for Christians, not for Jewish people," he continues.

Meanwhile, Elizabeth had asked her Christian friends to pray that her Jewish doctor friend would have an insatiable desire to keep reading and would not be able to put the Bible down.

After a few days, he decided to start reading the New Testament.

"When I read the Gospels, I was amazed!" Marc remembers. "Jesus was a Jew who came for the Jewish people. He lived a perfect life in regard to Torah (Jewish instruction), and He was our example. He died for our sins."

As he read the Gospel of John, the young doctor who thought he had everything realized he had nothing.

"I was convicted of the sinfulness of my lifestyle and knew what I had to do," he says. "I fell on my knees and I confessed my sins to God and asked Jesus, the promised Messiah, to come into my life."

God had spoken to him and revealed Himself just as Elizabeth had promised.

Shortly thereafter, Marc became a member of a Messianic Jewish congregation in Owings Mills, Maryland, where he could worship Jesus as Messiah in a distinctively Jewish way. He married the lifeguard named Elizabeth (who truly had been used to save his life).

A prestigious fellowship in arthritis and rheumatology research awaited him at Einstein and Montefiori in New York City, but he turned it down because he now felt God calling him as a new believer in a different direction, away from the culture of his youth.

He called up the National Health Service Corps and volunteered to work in an area with a shortage of physicians. The

NHSC accepted him, despite the fact that his request was very unusual: Corps members were not usually volunteers but *obligated* to work to pay back financial assistance received during medical school.

After some searching Marc found a position in Big Island, Virginia, in the Blue Ridge Mountains, where he practiced general internal and family medicine as the *only* physician in a twenty-mile area. His office was on top of the rescue-squad building, and he functioned as the area's "emergency-room" doctor, as the squad brought everybody to him first.

He and Elizabeth joined a small Baptist church, where he was touched by the people's down-to-earth lifestyle and their simple yet unshakable faith in the Lord.

He was also touched by some of his patients with cancer, who had to travel hours to the nearest medical center for research protocols. Even the closest oncologist was a forty-minute drive over windy roads through the mountains.

God was about to use these circumstances to change yet again the direction of this young doctor's life. Marc began giving some experimental chemotherapy in his office because it was too far for patients to go back and forth to medical centers.

He developed growing interest in treating cancer, and at God's leading, he left his rural practice after seven years to become a specialist in oncology. After completing two years of training at Hershey Medical Center, Marc and Elizabeth and their two young daughters began to search for the right town for him to open a private practice. They both thought something warm down south in the Carolinas or Virginia would be nice. Elizabeth especially wanted to be near the ocean. They looked into several positions, but nothing was working out.

Meanwhile Marc was driving forty miles from Hershey each month to the small town of Hanover because Hanover Hospital needed an oncologist at its tumor board meetings. None of the Hershey professors wanted to do it because they would have to get up so early to be in Hanover by 7 A.M.

But the hospital offered a couple hundred dollars for the monthly trek, and Marc agreed to do it because he needed to keep up with double house payments since their Virginia home had not sold. Within a year the offer came from Hanover Hospital to set him up in private practice in their community.

At first he and Elizabeth weren't interested, but soon they realized the town was only an hour from her parents in Baltimore and just forty-five minutes from the Messianic Jewish congregation where they had first worshiped together after he had come to faith in Messiah.

"We realized this was where we should be and where God wanted us to be," Marc says.

So in July 1989 Marc opened his private practice as the only oncologist in Hanover, Pennsylvania, a community of about fifteen thousand—the closest body of water being the Codorus Creek, which did run through his backyard!

Ever since coming here, Marc has tried to incorporate his faith and prayers into his medical practice and has at times even shared the gospel with patients. But there were so many hurts, fears, and needs in patients who were struggling with cancer and undergoing chemotherapy that he barely had time to scratch the surface.

Then in May 1990 he met me, when I was a newspaper reporter writing an article on the local hospital's new cancer support group. Six weeks later, ironically, I was back in his office as a patient with Stage III colon cancer. Over the next few years, Marc often referred patients to the Cancer Prayer Support Group I had started, and I often stopped by the chemo room to chat with friends receiving treatments.

But Marc knew this wasn't enough.

"On a day-to-day basis in my practice, I knew we still were not meeting the intense emotional and spiritual needs of patients," he says. Marc wanted someone who could work with the patients on a daily basis and offered me the job of patient advocate.

As a patient advocate I meet and greet the new patients as they enter the practice. I briefly relate my personal experience as one who had cancer, surgery, and chemotherapy, and I offer to discuss emotional and spiritual questions, while providing encouragement and support throughout patients' treatments. I am available to talk, pray, laugh, and cry with patients and their families, and my services are available free to *any* area cancer patients.

Most cancer patients experience distress, fear, and questions after being diagnosed with a life-threatening illness. I have instant credibility because I have "been there."

My job is to provide a biblical perspective on their questions and to point them to the "God of all hope." I pray for them and *with* them every chance I get. (We even have designated one of the metal flags outside the examining rooms as a "prayer flag," and if it's up, it means I'm praying with a patient and Marc waits to come in.)

"Having a patient advocate makes so much sense that I wonder why we didn't do it sooner," he told me shortly after I started working with him, adding that he "can't imagine" practicing medicine without having someone in a position like mine.

I can't imagine what my life would be like *without* being a patient advocate. It's incredible to me what one small prayer of thankfulness has led to.

If you have a cancer diagnosis, I'm wondering if you have found anything for which to be thankful in the midst of your circumstances. You probably don't have a Messianic Jewish oncologist (if you do, we'd love to know!), but I believe there is something or someone for which you can say a prayer of thanks. It may be just the prayer God wants to use to begin to bless your life.

Go ahead, be thankful in all things, even in cancer.

Be encouraged: A prayer of thanksgiving can unleash the power of God because He is able to do far more than we can ask or imagine.

The Heart, Mind, and Soul
of a Cancer Survivor

I DON'T KNOW what your attitude was like when somebody
smacked you with the words "you have cancer," but I didn't
have a very good attitude about my diagnosis. It didn't make
any sense to me. I hadn't even had a cold for four years. There
was no cancer in my family anywhere—certainly not colon
cancer, which normally strikes people sixty-five and older.
(Only about 5 percent of the new cases are in people under
forty.)

The doctors shook their heads and said I had done everything right *not* to get cancer. I never said it aloud, but in my
heart I said, *Why me?* I remember looking around at others
who were not taking good care of themselves and thinking,
This person should have cancer, or *That person should have
cancer. I shouldn't have it.*

As I already mentioned, my feelings were complicated by
the fact that my husband's first wife had died of Lou Gehrig's
disease while they were newlyweds in 1971. *Dear God,* my
heart cried out, *he's already buried one wife; surely this cannot
be happening again. . . . Why me?*

And then one day I was having lunch with my friend Pat
whom I had met at the hospital's cancer support group. She
had non-Hodgkin's lymphoma and was telling me that she
never asked, "Why me?"

Instead she asked, "Why not me?"

I was incredulous, but she was very serious. I began to think about her words. *Why not me?*

I knew the statistics—about one out of three people will eventually get cancer—but somehow I was positive I would be one of the ones who didn't. Somehow I had convinced myself that if I was a good person and did the right things, I would be guaranteed not to have any suffering. I would never have spoken that hypothesis out loud—it sounded much too vain—but in reality that's what I was saying when I said, "Why me?" I was projecting the notion that somehow bad things don't happen to good people.

We all know that's not true. Throughout this book, I've introduced you to some really wonderful people who had to face cancer. In fact, some of the *nicest* people I've ever met have cancer.

So I have been forced to admit that in this world filled with sickness and disease, I am not immune. I did my best not to "get" cancer, but it didn't work.

As I walked this journey with an unwanted, unwelcome disease, both in my own life and in the lives of hundreds of cancer patients, I began to ask myself, *What does the heart, mind, and soul of a cancer survivor need?*

This chapter is my answer to that question for myself. Perhaps it will be the answer for you, as well.

~ ~ ~

The heart of a cancer survivor needs to find the right attitude.

Remember how I said I didn't have a very good attitude when I was diagnosed with cancer?

Well, I finally got to the point—and I know many of you made it there much faster than I did—where I asked, *Why not me?*

Acceptance, I believe, is the first step necessary in moving your heart toward the right attitude.

It's often said that there are two kinds of people in life: optimists and pessimists. I want to remind you that optimism will not always change the inevitable. Take the case of the optimist who fell out of the twelfth-story window. As he went by the fifth story, he looked around, smiled, and said to himself, "So far, so good."

Pessimism isn't a very good idea either.

Did you hear about the farmer who lived next door to a pessimist? If the farmer said, "Isn't it a beautiful sunny day?" the pessimist would reply, "We need rain." If it rained and the farmer commented on how wonderful it was to have rain, the pessimist would reply, "It'll probably ruin the crops." He always managed to see the worst in any situation.

But one day the farmer decided he would put an end to his neighbor's pessimism. He called his neighbor to come over and see an amazing trick his dog could do. The farmer proceeded to throw a stick out into the middle of his pond. Immediately the dog jumped toward the pond and walked on *top* of the water out to the floating stick. He carefully picked it up in his mouth, walked back across the top of the water safely to the shore, and laid the stick at the pessimist's feet.

The farmer looked at his neighbor and said, "Pretty amazing, huh?" to which the pessimist replied, "Can't swim, can he?"

You probably think I'm going to tell you to be an optimist. I am not.

I have found that the best attitude for a cancer patient is neither total optimism (*without a doubt, I'm going to be cured*) nor total pessimism (*without a doubt, I'm going to die*), but realism (*without a doubt, I have a life-threatening illness and I may or may not get better, so I will plan for both*).

When we insist that we are going to be cured, we set ourselves up for a terrible defeat if that doesn't happen. On the other hand, if we insist that our situation is hopeless, we already are defeated before we start. I believe it's best to be realistic and make plans to be financially, emotionally, and spiritually ready to depart this life. That's not giving up. It's coming to grips with our own mortality, so we really can live life fully without fear of death.

I have seen scores of people who refuse to entertain the thought that they might not be cured of cancer because they wanted to remain totally optimistic. Those who weren't cured were devastated. I also know scores of people whose situation was medically hopeless, but they continued to live life fully and some of them even went on to become cancer-free! (Just this week, a patient was in our office who relapsed only three months after she had a bone marrow transplant for non-Hodgkin's lymphoma. Because there was no other treatment at that time that could offer her the hope of a cure, she simply had the cancerous lump removed and did nothing else. That was eight years ago, and there has never been another sign of the cancer!)

Please don't misunderstand me, but I feel there is a difference between total optimism and a positive attitude. Total optimism says, "I'm absolutely, positively going to be cured." A positive attitude says, "I hope and pray and even expect that I'm going to be cured, but even if I'm not, I will not be defeated."

A totally optimistic attitude insists lemons will get sweeter. A positive attitude makes lemonade out of the lemons.

A positive attitude will help heal you—physically, emotionally, and spiritually—but it may or may not cure you. As a cancer-support-group facilitator and a cancer patient advocate, I've seen plenty of people with wonderful, positive attitudes who didn't get better and I've seen people with crummy attitudes doing quite well. I wish I could say that if you just have a positive attitude you'll get better, but there is no such guarantee. If we're honest, we all must admit that we have known people with great attitudes who did not get well from cancer or myriad other illnesses.

I remember when people used to say to me, "Think positive; you can beat this." That really didn't make me feel better. Instead I felt more pressure. If I wasn't positive and optimistic enough, I wasn't going to get better and it would be all my fault.

I've since come to realize that being positive and having a good attitude changes us and those around us for the better, but it is not a guarantee that we will get better physically.

There were many days I shed tears and many days I held little private pity parties for myself, but I did try to take control of my heart's attitude. So much else was out of my control:

What chemo drugs I needed
How often I needed to take them
What their toxicity was
What my medical prognosis was

I had no control over any of those, but I could control my attitude. Having the right attitude will definitely give you better quality of life and perhaps more quantity.

I love how author Chuck Swindoll describes the importance of attitude: "Words can never adequately convey the incredible impact of our attitude toward life. The longer I live the more convinced I become that life is 10 percent what happens to us and 90 percent how we respond to it. I believe the single most significant decision I can make on a day-to-day basis is my choice of attitude. It is more important than my past, my education, my bankroll, my successes or failures, fame or pain, what other people think of me or say about me, my circumstances, or my position. Attitude keeps me going or cripples my progress. It alone fuels my fire or assaults my hope. When my attitudes are right, there's no barrier too high, no valley too deep, no dream too extreme, no challenge too great for me."[1]

The heart of a cancer survivor—your heart—needs to find the right attitude.

~ ~ ~

The mind of a cancer survivor needs to find peace.

Before I had cancer I really wasn't much of a worrier. When people would tell me they were worried about something, I would very *sensitively* tell them, "Well, just don't think about it."

After my diagnosis, I became a professional worrier. It's hard not to be paranoid when people are always feeling you for lumps and checking you for recurrences.

At one point shortly after I finished my chemo I found a lump on my neck. (This came soon after I talked with a friend who had had thyroid cancer.) I kept pressing on this lump, and sure enough, it got sorer and sorer. When I went for my next recheck with Marc, I mentioned the sore lump. He politely told me, "Quit pressing on the lump or you will die. You're pressing on your carotid artery and you're cutting off the blood supply to your brain!"

I worried about other things, like my husband being widowed again and my daughters growing up without a mother. I worried that each holiday was my last and that I would never feel normal again. I knew it wasn't good to worry, so I worried because I worried so much.

But it's hard to stop worrying.

I remember the first day I didn't worry about cancer. I was a newspaper reporter at the time and engrossed in a story I was writing on my laptop. All of a sudden I looked at my watch with amazement—I had gone a whole two hours without thinking about cancer.

That was the beginning of my learning the secret of not worrying: something else had to occupy my mind. Philippians 4:8 says, "Finally, brothers, whatever is true, whatever is noble, whatever is right, whatever is pure, whatever is lovely, whatever is admirable—if anything is excellent or praiseworthy—think about such things" (NIV).

When other thoughts came into my mind, worrisome thoughts, I asked myself if they fit these criteria: true, noble, right, pure, lovely, admirable, excellent, or praiseworthy. If not, I pushed them out and replaced them with a thought that did. For me it was usually one of God's promises from His

Word. When you want to empty your mind of worry, make sure you find something encouraging to put in its place.

Another way to combat worrying is not to look too far down the road. Holocaust survivor Corrie ten Boom wrote, "Worrying about tomorrow robs today of its joy." That is so true.

Your mind finds peace when you live in the present and not in the "what-ifs" of the future. People used to say to me, "Just take one day at a time." Personally, I couldn't think about taking one day a time. That was way too much. At first I only thought about taking one *hour* at a time.

Thinking about facing six months of chemotherapy or thirty days of radiation or years of follow-ups can seem way too overwhelming. Thinking about just getting through today's chemo or today's radiation is a far better choice.

I believe getting through treatments is a lot like athletic training. I started jogging in the summer of 1998. I'm not sure what possessed me to do this. I was forty-four at the time and had never jogged in my adult life (unless you count the times I ran after the school bus when I didn't have my kids out the door on time).

But I started jogging in August 1998, after we returned from a relaxing vacation. I am not a morning person, but I got up at 6:30 every other day and ran two miles in the Pigeon Hills, where I live.

My children, then sixteen, eighteen, and twenty, were incredulous when I started doing this. They asked a lot of questions:

Why is Mom buying running shoes?
She runs?
In the morning?
She gets up before Dad?
***Our* mom?**

I really don't even like running; the only part that feels good is when I stop. (Although I've learned since I started running on an indoor track at the YMCA that I don't hate running, I hate hills!) All along the way I have to talk myself into not quitting.

See that telephone pole up there? You can make it, I say. *You've done this before, you can do it again. Remember you get tomorrow off; you don't have to do this again right away.*

I especially have to talk myself into making it up the huge hill to my house. When I first started I said I would never be able to make the hill, but one day I decided just to run up the top half, which wasn't so steep. Another day I had just reached the bottom and was ready to start walking when I saw my neighbor Jim sitting in his car at the bottom of the hill waiting for his kids' bus. Jim is younger than I am and very athletic, and I knew he would give me a hard time if he saw me stop and walk up the hill, so I kept running . . . and I made it.

It's the same way I talked myself into going in for a chemo treatment every week for six months.

You've done this before; you can do it again.
Remember, afterward you have six days off.
Forget about all the times still to come.
Don't look at the big hill.
Just focus on what you're doing right now.

As long as I kept my mind in the present, focused on that goal, I had peace.

When you hear the phrase *what if* pop into your mind, you know peace is about to leave you. About 90 percent of the things I worried about never came true. Most of the "what-ifs" never happened.

In April 1997 I was faced with a possible "what-if." For me, my big "what-if" is, "What if the cancer comes back?" (Colon cancer normally cannot be cured if it recurs, because it usually has spread to vital organs.)

That April an episode of irregular vaginal bleeding led to a sonogram, which showed a growth wrapped around my ovary.

"Probably just a benign cyst"—which I have a history of.
"We'll watch it for three months," my gynecologist said, and I
agreed. But a couple of days later, she called me back at work.

"I discussed your case with my colleagues, and they all feel
this is an abnormal growth and it needs to come out," she said.

"What do you think it is?" I asked.

"Probably nothing," she said, "but it could be ovarian
cancer or a recurrence of the colon cancer." I felt my stomach
tightening. I tried to remain calm and nonchalant.

"We'll need to have a general surgeon on hand in case it is a
colon recurrence and you need more surgery," she added. We
went over pre-op details and I hung up.

All of the worries and fears I thought I had conquered after
almost seven years were back.

In my job as patient advocate I encourage patients emotionally and spiritually, reminding them that God can be trusted
no matter what the circumstances. Now I would find out again
if I could trust Him in spite of *my* circumstances.

It took me about forty-eight hours, but I remember sitting
in my bedroom and saying to God, "Okay, I don't like this one
bit. I think it stinks. I don't want to die and I don't want to go
through more chemo. But God, You have proven Yourself so
faithful in my life and have blessed me so much through my
cancer experience, I would be nuts not to trust You now. So,
whatever is ahead, I know You are in control and I trust You."

Peace immediately flooded my mind. (P.S. The tumor was
benign.)

I read somewhere and firmly believe that "sorrow looks
back, worry looks around, and faith looks up."

The mind of a cancer survivor—your mind—needs to find
peace.

Finally, the soul of a cancer survivor needs to find hope.
I think the biggest thing that most of us cancer patients

want is hope—hope for today and especially hope for the tomorrows.

We hope for a cure or at least a long remission. We hope the surgery is successful or the treatment isn't too toxic. I've seen people put their hope in all sorts of things—vitamins, nutritional supplements, macrobiotic diets, coffee enemas. Some people put their hope in their doctor and his or her abilities. Some people feel they have no hope. Maybe some physician has even told you there *is* no hope.

I like what Marc tells people when they ask, "Is there any hope?"

"There's always hope in God," he says.

I recently read a piece on hope and I like how it explains that hope doesn't have to be singular:

> Hope comes naturally to some people. Others may have to work to achieve it. Acquiring information, gaining control, developing faith, setting priorities, finding a sense of purpose—all these are ways of getting in touch with hope.
>
> When most patients say "hope," they mean the hope of a cure. To us, hope means much more than that. We define hope as a positive attitude, not necessarily related to achieving a cure. Hope means accepting the reality of any situation but focusing on the redeeming aspects of that situation. To hope is to look for the positive in one's circumstances, whether those circumstances are good or bad. . . . To hope is to be able to focus on what matters the most to you. This means that hope is highly individual. . . . For one person, hope might be the hope of a cure. For another, it might be the hope of a peaceful death.
>
> For one person, hope might be hope for the highest possible quality of life. For another, it might be the hope of bringing life to a positive completion—by mending old

quarrels, by finishing work left undone, by coming to terms with old fears.

For one person, hope might be the hope of living in such a way that one's life has made a difference to others. For another, it might be the hope of dying in such a way that one's death has made a difference to others.[2]

When I was going through my treatments for cancer and then living with the reality that I had maybe a 40 percent chance of surviving cancer, many people asked me, "How do you do it?" The answer was that I had hope. Nothing about my cancer made any sense to me.

Why should I, a young, healthy person have cancer?
Why should my husband have to face the possibility of being widowed again?
How could my three girls grow up without their mother?
None of it made sense.

Only one thing did make sense and that was knowing that this life is not all there is—that if at age thirty-six, I was to die from cancer (or anything else) I knew where I was going to spend eternity because of my personal relationship with God through His Son, Jesus.

Life was not being fair to me, but God would be. He had provided a way for my salvation. I could go to heaven—where Scripture promises there are no more tears, no more sickness, and no more dying (Revelation 21:4). I was not getting short-changed by dying young, because this life is not all there is. Now that made sense and gave me hope.

The more I trusted in the Lord, the more hope I had. Romans 15:13 came true in my life as never before: "May the God of hope fill you with all joy and peace as you trust in him, so that you may overflow with hope by the power of the Holy Spirit" (NIV).

The soul of a cancer survivor—your soul—needs to find hope.

~ ~ ~

Dear friend, I wish you well on your—or your loved
  one's—journey with cancer.
I wish you a heart that has found the right attitude—a
  positive, realistic attitude.
I wish you a mind that has found peace—by replacing
  worries with better thoughts and by focusing on the
  present and not on the "what-ifs" of the future.
And I wish you a soul that has found hope—a hope based
  on the God of all Creation, who gives life true meaning.

God *can* make blessing come from cancer when God and
cancer meet, but we have to let Him choose the blessing. Every
person in this book received a blessing from cancer, but it
wasn't always the one they might have chosen. And sometimes, as the saying goes, when they couldn't see God's hand,
they simply trusted His heart. Psalm 50:15 says, "Trust me in
your times of trouble, and I will rescue you, and you will give
me glory" (NLT).

On the fifth anniversary of my cancer surgery, I wrote the
following poem summing up what my journey with cancer has
taught me:

> *When your world is crashing down around you, trust Him.*
> *When what is unfolding doesn't make sense, trust Him.*
> *When you see no light at the end of the tunnel, trust Him.*
> *When your silent tears spill down, trust Him.*
> *When the pain refuses to subside, trust Him.*
> *When your heart screams, "Why?" trust Him.*
> *When you have more questions than answers, trust Him.*
> *When the devil tells you otherwise, trust Him.*

When it's the last thing you feel like doing, trust Him.
When there's simply nothing else to do, trust Him.

Be encouraged: God can be trusted in all things . . . even cancer.

endnotes

CHAPTER 2: Close Encounters of the Divine Kind
[1] Mrs. Charles E. Cowman, *Streams in the Desert,* vol. 2 (Grand Rapids, Mich.: Zondervan, 1966).

CHAPTER 4: When God Did the Heimlich Maneuver
[1] Philip Yancey, *Disappointment with God* (Grand Rapids, Mich.: Zondervan, 1988), 182–184.
[2] Ibid., 170.

CHAPTER 7: "It was our first prayer together"
[1] David Biebel, *If God Is So Good, Why Do I Hurt So Bad?* (Grand Rapids, Mich.: Fleming H. Revell, a division of Baker Book House, 1989), 15.

CHAPTER 19: The Heart, Mind, and Soul of a Cancer Survivor
[1] Charles R. Swindoll, *Strengthening Your Grip* (Nashville, Tenn.: W Publishing Group, formerly Word Publishing, 1982), pp. 206–207. Used by permission of Insight for Living (the Bible-teaching ministry of Charles R. Swindoll), Plano, TX 75025. All rights reserved.
[2] Brent G. Ryder, *The Alpha Book on Cancer and Living* (Alameda, Ca.: The Alpha Institute, 1993), 392–393.

**WHEN WE FIRST FACE THE DISEASE,
GOD IS THERE.**

**WHEN WE CONTINUE TO LIVE
IN ITS SHADOW . . .
GOD IS STILL THERE.**

Another inspiring
book from
Lynn Eib

*Finding the Light
in Cancer's Shadow*

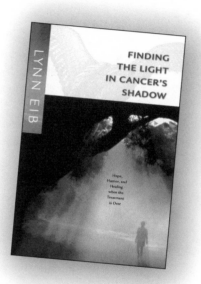

Cancer survivors often continue living
in the shadow of the disease—whether
they're in treatment, remission, or
facing a recurrence.

Finding the Light in Cancer's Shadow
is an amazing book about finding
hope, faith, and true wholeness in the
aftermath of cancer.

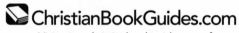ChristianBookGuides.com

Visit www.christianbookguides.com for
a discussion guide and other book-group resources
for When God & Cancer Meet.